Only You, Christine, Only You!

Christine Komoroski-McCohnell

iUniverse, Inc.
New York   Bloomington

Only You, Christine, Only You!

iUniverse books may be ordered through booksellers or by contacting:

iUniverse
1663 Liberty Drive
Bloomington, IN 47403
www.iuniverse.com
1-800-Authors (1-800-288-4677)

ISBN: 978-1-4401-3092-2 (sc)
ISBN: 978-1-4401-3093-9 (ebook)
ISBN: 978-1-4401-3094-6 (dj)

Printed in the United States of America

iUniverse rev. date: 10/07/2009

Contents

"The roots of a lotus are in the mud, the stem grows up through the water, and the heavily scented flower lies pristinely above the water, basking in the sunlight. This pattern of growth signifies the progress of the soul from the primeval mud of materialism, through the waters of experience, and into the bright sunshine of enlightenment." http://www.religionfacts.com/buddhism/symbols/lotus.htm

Christine Komoroski-McCohnell's *Only You, Christine, Only You!* describes a young woman's coming of age in contemporary America. Memoirs are flooding the marketplace, and it would be easy to dismiss this work as one more exercise in narcissism. Potential readers who choose that option are depriving themselves of the opportunity to participate, almost viscerally, in a life affirming transcendent tale.

Her journey is marked by constant physical and emotional pain from birth, but it is also the journey of a soul who never surrendered her autonomy as a person to the omnipresent obstacles of Cerebral Palsy. She speaks in the voice of the "different" child and woman, and in so doing she gives voice to all those who are labeled and judged because of their "difference." This voice is raw with anger. This voice is reflective and frequently quite funny. Her metaphor of a "staircase of oppression" symbolizes the struggle of all people, not just those categorized as disabled, in all times and places, to be included and treated as full and equal members of their communities.

Komoroski-McCohnell has another voice. She speaks to us as a scholar and teacher. She draws upon her training as a counselor. Perhaps most valuable is her ability to mesh scholarship and life experience to illuminate our understanding of how disabled people perceive themselves, and how the attitudes of the abled magnify difference.

She speaks as a complex, difficult, imperfect human being. She struggles not to be defined or confined by her disability, and she struggles to embrace it as a significant part of her personhood, but only one part. The routine issues any of us have to deal with are hers too, but always refracted through the prism of the CP. In recounting her life, Christine takes us on an unexpected *tour d'horizon* of contemporary America. She transcends her personal story as she discusses family, class, race, sexuality, and identity as both limits and opportunities. This unexpected dimension lifts this memoir into a different category. In sharing her story with us, Christine Komoroski-McCohnell holds up a mirror in which we all are reflected.

Her story is one of incredible courage, commitment, and most importantly, of love. Love sought. Love freely given, received, and requited. Christine is the bravest person I have ever known. I count it an honor to be her colleague and friend. She is a lotus in our midst.

Mike Fluhr
Professor of Political Science, Ramapo College of New Jersey

This book is dedicated with love to my Mom,
who encouraged me from Day One;
as well as to all the other wonderful, colorful,
peaceful people in my life!

Prologue

The purpose of this memoir is to re-live my life and, by so doing, I
hope to share some wisdom with the reader.

My story is not a Hallmark story. Like most people with disabilities,
I do not fit some ideal standard of morality; rather, I am a human
being with both flaws and good qualities.

This is a story of interest to folks
that really want to learn about the life of one woman with CP.

This story is like a staircase; you will understand why as you come
and climb it with me.

To protect privacy and identity I've changed some names.

My Childhood

As I awaken this morning, I feel utterly depleted and don't want to see the outside world. My CP (cerebral palsy) kept me up all night with nonstop coughing. Shit. Why does Mac, my fiancé have to take a shower so early in the morning? In a few minutes, he'll parade out of the bathroom, singing about how resplendent this day is gonna be. How does he know that it's gonna be a great day? It's pouring rain outside, dammit. I feel like shit, and he's proclaiming that it's gonna be a dazzling day?!

Mac calls to me, "Honey, what time are you leaving for your office today?"

"I'm leaving the house around ten o'clock."

Mac knows he shouldn't ask me any questions before coffee, but you gotta love a sexy man, my gorgeous fiancé, with his beautiful body and calm repose that melts my soul. In so many ways, he is the epitome of my other half, the polar opposite of my hyper self. Yin and yang. Black and white. We are one wonderful fit. During passionate lovemaking, when he's inside of me, that's the time I feel most complete.

I can't imagine how my mother felt when I was inside of her. Right now, I feel achy and bloated. Maybe being pregnant might be a hundred times worse; however, my mom told me that she felt her best when she was pregnant. I don't think she felt her best *delivering* me because I was weighing in an unfathomed fourteen pounds at birth.

While Mac is yodeling about how marvelous this rainy day is, we'll just ignore him and Let's fast forward to the day of my birth, March 9ᵗʰ, 1974. My mom was a diabetic, which led to my weight growing the closer she got to delivery. The doctor had told her that there was no need for a Caesarian so she had me naturally, vaginally. Due to major complications in the birth canal, I entered the world with trouble ahead. I often wonder if maybe I ate too much as an embryo! Well, I'm in the world now, so let's move on from my dietary dilemma (although to this day, I'm still conscious of my weight!).

When I came into the world, it was a scenario much different from the typical, loving introduction between mother and infant. As we all know, when mother and child unite for the first time, they begin to bond within seconds. My mom and I had a totally remote experience. Remote? Indeed. I was taken away without my mom even seeing me, and she was promptly put to sleep. There was no peaceful introduction here. I was whisked away in an ambulance to a nearby hospital, while my mother was placed on a floor away from the nursery. The doctor believed that it would help her to not see other parents and infants and become emotional. My mother told me she knew something was wrong when she woke up and saw an old woman next to her in her room.

In several conversations with Mom, she has been hesitant to talk about this time in her life. I respect her hesitancy to rehash these memories, considering the painful trauma she endured. All I know are a few recreated conversations that went on between the doctor and my parents. I'll call him Doctor X.

I want you to know that the year I was born, 1974, was three years before regulations for *The Rehabilitation Act of 1973* were passed, which then made this important law enforceable. What important law? I add that question because it amazes me how many people know nothing about *The Rehabilitation Act*. It's especially crucial for parents and caregivers of school-age kids with disabilities to be familiar with this groundbreaking legislation. Also called 504 legislation, this vital precursor to *The Americans with Disabilities Act* states that all government agencies must be completely accessible for people with disabilities. Completely–as in providing accessibility for any reasonable

2

disability accommodation you can think of. Anyway, the regulations were not passed until 1977, so the general mentality of doctors was different when I was born.

Since I was born with pronounced CP, Doctor X advised my mom, "You have three beautiful kids; don't stretch yourself out with Christine. Put her in an institution, and go on with your life, Teresa." I guess Mom had formed a strong, loving bond with me while I was inside her. She completely dismissed the doctor's advice.

When my spirited mother was released from the hospital five days afterward, she finally went to see her big baby girl. I just realized while writing this that I love to stay in hotels. My very first "hotel" was Beth Israel Hospital in Newark, New Jersey. My "extended stay" lasted three months. Maybe I owe Doctor X some gratitude for my love of relaxing vacations at extended-stay hotels. Anyway, I kindly allowed my mom to visit me at my hotel. I was in an incubator, and my mom told me that she cried to my father because I was too big for the little space. My parents never mistook me in the ICU, because the teeny neighbors on either side of me weighed about one pound each. So, I guess my size was actually a positive thing.

Still today, I get tears in my eyes when my mom tells me she visited me every day until I came home. I'm thinking to myself, "Why did she bother driving to Newark, when I really didn't know she was there?" I mean, I had my teeny, tiny friends, and she had three big kids back in Scotch Plains. I'm not a mother yet, but a proud stepmom-to-be, so I really don't understand the motherly instinct to the fullest. Of course, my devoted daddy always came after a long day at work to see me, as well. My parents were loving and stalwart from the start.

Another story that I heard, through my mom's sister was that, due to my size, I was raising hell right from the beginning. Let me explain why. Did you ever go shopping in an infant department? You'll notice that the sizes are very distinct: zero to three months, three months to six months, and so on. The first sleeper pajama that my mom hugged me in was an eighteen-month size, and I was two months old! Prior to that, I had been hooked up to wires and machines, wearing only a diaper. My aunt, who hardly ever plans ahead, had bought my mom baby clothes for me, all three- to six-month size. Needless to say, she was upset that her planned purchases had not worked out.

3

My next oldest sibling was six and a half years old at the time of my birth. Busy with a trio of other kids, my mom chose to simply order a big basket of clothes for me. The local department store said to her, "Just call so we know the sex of the baby." My mom called and told them that I was a really big, bouncing baby girl. They asked my mom twice what my weight was, obviously shocked by the answer.

When I was three months old, the doctor informed my parents that I was ready to go home to meet my sister and two brothers. He also strongly recommended that they hire a live-in nanny to care for me because of the intensive 24/7 care I required. Picture this: I'm now a fifteen-pound baby drinking from an itsy-bitsy bottle, and my mom was elated if I drank two ounces in the course of an hour! You can imagine the kind of care I needed.

Back then, my father was not poor by any means; he was a successful businessman, but even he could not afford to turn our basement into living quarters for a nanny. Luckily, my grandfather agreed to help my parents so that there was a room for me. I imagine that I must have been excited to come home. My well-equipped nursery was in between my parents' room and my sister's room. To this day, my sister Kimberly says that I was the Nightmare Baby from Hell, because I took over the whole house and reigned supreme. During the day, I was the sweetest infant you'd ever want to meet, but during the night, I was a terror. I used to scream my head off from 7 pm until 2 am every night, like clockwork. I'm sure that everyone in the house had a little problem with me. If you think about it, I was a pretty smart infant: My parents had visited me in the hospital during the day, and I was so sweet to them that they yearned to take me home. They had not known that my true colors flamed at night.

On a more serious note, I'm sure my development was in chaos. I'm not an MD, but my personal opinion is that infants don't have it easy as they are developing a whole new soul in a body and world that is unknown to them. So when someone says *all* a baby does is eat a lot, sleep a lot, and poop a lot, think again.

When I came home, my maternal grandmother was very involved with my care. My parents hired a nanny/housekeeper, but my grandmother was always hesitant to have an outsider take care of her "special" granddaughter. One day my grandma pulled up to our

4

house while my mom was picking up my siblings from school. As she approached my nursery, Grandma found all of the housekeepers on the block in my room, praying. One was on the floor because "the Spirit" was in her. My grandma was horrified. My mother walked into the house to hear Grandma yelling, "What are they doing up there?" My mom simply explained that they were trying to lift "the Curse" from me. Mom shrugged and said, "If it helps her get better, that's fine." I think my grandmother fired my first nanny about five times. After the first time, the stubborn nanny just ignored her and remained for years.

Mac is still singing away, and I'm debating exactly what material I'm going to use for tonight's lecture. I am an adjunct professor teaching Disability Studies at Ramapo College of New Jersey. Tonight's topic is one of my favorites, and also the one I have researched the most. Identity Formation has intrigued me ever since I was a senior at Ramapo College myself—when I was working with children with disabilities. I came to realize that they had not yet developed their identities, and I have seen how my own model of identity is markedly different now from what it was ten years ago as a college student. I guess it would be helpful if I define these identity models for you, huh?

The first model that I discuss in my class is the Minority Model. There are other models of identity formation, such as the Moral Model, the Medical Model, and the Affirmation Model. The Minority Model says that people with disabilities embrace their identity as a proud, independent population. They believe that the problem does not involve the person with the disability, but rather with society itself. For example, if a person in a wheelchair cannot get into a restaurant because there is no ramp, it is not the disabled person's fault; rather, it's the owner's fault for not having the proper access, or proper parking, or even large print menus, or accessible restrooms—whatever accommodation may be needed and required by law. People who identify with this model believe that attitudes are the real disabilities, and are usually very involved with the Disability Rights Movement and Disability Culture.

On the opposite end of the spectrum is the Moral Model, which believes that disability is either a gift from God or a curse from God. The supernatural is a strong force in this model. The predominant notion is feeling guilt toward the person with the disability, or feeling pity for that person. It might be confusing to you about how guilt ties in to people with disabilities, so I'll break it down for you. Take a child with a disability whose parents identify with the Moral Model, even if this is an unconscious state. The parents will say to themselves or to each other, "We must have done something *wrong* because God has given us a child with a disability." This example is the epitome of guilt, which can lead to a variety of results: abuse, punishment, neglect, or even "selfless" devotion to the child–so much so that the disabled person is not given the right of adulthood. Again, this behavior is motivated by guilt-ridden family members.

Another example of the Moral Model results in the following thinking: "We are two such special individuals that God has given us an angel; we must carry out our duty that was placed upon us by God. How can we make it up to this child?" This specific guilt trip results in infantilizing and overprotecting the child because parents are "dutifully" carrying out God's will and shielding their offspring. Or, as noted, it can result in grievous mistreatment and abuse because it is so painful for the parents to endure.

Or, another example is the cultural tradition of literally "beating the devil" out of people with disabilities. Severe corporal punishment is obviously abusive, but so too is overprotection. A disabled person who associates with the Moral Model might say: "Why me? What have I done wrong to acquire this disability?" (In fact, most disabilities *are* acquired, and not genetically inherited.) Independence is not in their vocabulary; they (sometimes unconsciously) expect pity and protection from outsiders and feel shame, as opposed to the Minority Model, which feels great pride and empowerment and seeks independence.

The Medical Model states that people with disabilities are desperately trying to achieve able-bodied status; in other words, they are looking for a *cure*. They say that they are empowered individuals with disabilities because they are so focused on researching and obtaining that cure. Often these individuals choose not to embrace the Disability Rights Movement and Disability Culture. They ignore the fact that they have a rich history behind them. They may not be totally aware of the progress that the disabled community has made over the last thirty years. In tying this back to my infancy, when the doctor told my family to institutionalize me, this exemplified the Medical Model–not concerned so much with trying to cure the baby (me), as to do away with it. He couldn't cure *me*, but he could "cure" the situation by disposing of me. Again, this model is exemplified when parents elect to abort disabled fetuses. For example, if a woman is carrying a Down syndrome baby or a fetus with spina bifida, the doctor will most likely ask, "Do you want to terminate the pregnancy?" It is obvious that the doctor and the medical community have great power over the disabled community, whether it is "cure 'em, kill 'em, or institutionalize 'em." The Medical Model disparages disability. It assumes that we are "less than" and undesirable. Cure, cure, cure is the primary motto. Full cultural inclusion and celebration are not considered, nor is it understood that many folks with disabilities are indeed proud of their disabled status. Disability Pride is not unlike Feminist Pride, or Black Pride, or Gay Pride, or Irish Pride, or Italian Pride, or any type of ethnic pride—for that matter, American Pride. I think you get my point. The Medical Model dispraises disabilities and Disability Pride.

The Affirmation Model, to me, is a combination of the Minority Model and the Medical Model. The Affirmation Model states that a positive identity comes from within. This model does not blame society's attitudes or the supernatural; it just identifies the concrete evidence that a person with a disability is experiencing. I'll give you an example of the Affirmation Model: I have CP, and I also teach a Disability Studies course. I am an empowered, working woman of the New Millennium. Yet I often get angry at my "impairment" and I sometimes disparage it myself. However, *I do not want a cure or pity*, because I live in a rich culture that the disabled community has provided for me. On any given day, I do not embrace or feel proud of the physical pain that I experience. The fatigue that I encounter is stressful on the day following a long day at the office. I'm sometimes exhausted in the morning due to my respiratory condition that keeps Mac and me up all night. Needless to say, he's exhausted, too. I feel under pressure due to society's expectations, and I often become angry at those expectations because I cannot compete on the same level as able-bodied people. Nevertheless, I remain an empowered, accomplished, independent woman. Minority and Medical Models combined am I—a living example of the Affirmation Model. This model has provided me with a sense of belonging and has helped me to remember, to analyze, and to be at peace with life's arduous hurdles, which I refer to symbolically as "steps in the staircase of oppression" in my life. This staircase is my ever-present through-line.

Since I'm still debating what I'm going to lecture on tonight, maybe I'll just use these notes about the four models of Identity Formation in the disabled community. Believe it or not, Mac is still mid-chorus. I love him, but he doesn't sing as beautifully as my maternal grandmother.

One of my very first memories was my grandmother singing to me while she was watching me sleep in the crib. She had no idea that I was admiring her voice. She had no idea that I would be able to recall my babyhood, but I do remember. I would give anything to tell her how her voice soothed me. My grandma passed away recently, and my grandfather passed away several years ago. In telling my story, I am realizing what a loving impact these two individuals had on my infancy. My grandma *always* sang to me and had a unique touch in caring for me.

My grandma and my mother were very similar. I remember sitting with each of them in the rocking chair in my nursery, cradled in their arms. My mom had a mole on her face that I always had to touch in order to fall asleep. Thinking about that actually brings comfort to my soul. There is nothing like a mother's or a grandmother's security, and I treasured both generations of undying, indestructible female love.

I remember the Carter presidential election clearly (I was two years old) because on that day the housekeeper Doreen was holding me. Doreen was no substitute for Mommy or my grandma. My parents came in from voting, and I vividly remember Doreen's yellow uniform. I also remember my dad proudly saying, "We want Carter!" Doreen was the only housekeeper I remember, and that distinct memory is couched in the context of family and good feelings. It was genuinely the beginning of my awareness of social policy legislation that would affect me, positively and profoundly.

In that same period, I remember my first preschool. I attended the CP Center of Edison. As you can tell, Mom and I had this tremendous bond. She would take me to the CP Center for therapy and playgroups. While I was in the playgroup, she was in classes learning how to take care of her baby with CP. When we were separated, everyone in the

Center knew it because I screamed my head off! I clearly remember the playpen they plunked me in when I screamed.

Luckily, my mother met Lorraine, who became a very dear friend. They would sit together during their parenting classes, accompanied by the beautiful melody of my screaming. My mom would remark, "There goes Christine again." I hope she realizes that I took after her–because she'd always talk with Lorraine way too much and consequently got kicked out of her class while I got kicked out of playgroup. Like mother, like daughter. After several "detentions," we both got serious about my progress.

The CP Center taught me the essential tools I needed to function: walking, talking, eating, and more. The learning process wasn't easy, but my parents always wanted me to excel in anything I did. To appreciate the process, I'll tell you some stories that will help you understand why these basic skills were major accomplishments for me.

I had my very first boyfriend at age three and a half. I remember him absolutely lucidly. At this time, we were not able to talk, but we communicated *very* well. We could hug; we could smile; we could sit next to each other. I also remember the big, preschool room and trying to put beads on a string. (Today I still can't put beads on a string, but I *am* a professor. So there!) I vividly remember the speech room. They were teaching my mom how to stimulate my mouth muscles to suck on a bottle. I was sucking on the bottle until the age of four. I remember that because my brother Stevie would take my bottle away from me while he changed what I was watching on TV, the wonderful *Magic Garden*, to whatever he wanted to watch. He was very mean to me back then.

After becoming a pro at sucking, they wanted me to start chewing and stop sucking my table food. That was the first time I was rebellious. (Can you blame me? I just figured out sucking!) I recall sitting in front of the mirror with a Happy Meal in front of me and having the speech therapist, Travis, say to my mom, "Take the hamburger, and put it in her mouth." Then he said to me rather sternly, "Take little bites, Christine, and then chew." I took a little bite and proceeded to suck on the hamburger. "No, Christine, chew!" Well, I did not chew; I spat the hamburger right out into Travis's face. Needless to say, I went into "detention" again–they put me in the damn corner.

At home, I didn't get a break either. Gabrielle, my occupational therapist, came to work with me. My mom reports that I was a cute kid when the speech therapist, Jeanne, visited; she played with me and succumbed completely to my spoiled behavior. However, Gabrielle, the occupational therapist, was completely different from the rest of my growing team of caregivers. She did not give in to my adorable antics; she meant business. In fact, she was a regular Nurse Ratched. Despite my reactions to her, she was the one who taught me how to climb up stairs and feed myself. She and my mom designed the most uncomfortable wheelchair you could ever imagine, to keep me from settling into it and not making the effort to walk. Nurse Ratched also designed a standing table where I would stand and "play games" with her. I really hated her, and I would scream my head off for my mommy to rescue me from her.

Uh-oh! Mac has stopped singing. Have I left something messy in our bathroom? What have I done? With my absent-minded professor mentality, it could be anything. Let's see what he wants.

"Baby, are you listening to me?" he asks.

"Yes, dear. I heard everything you sang and said." I really hadn't. How am I gonna get out of this one? "I'm leaving the house for campus at about ten o'clock."

"What are you talking about? See, you don't listen to me. But I love you anyway. I said, 'If we go out for dinner, what about Thai food tonight?'"

"Sure, whatever you want, honey. But I leave the office a little before nine o'clock, so it'll be a late dinner."

I'm sure you don't wanna hear all the logistics about dinner, and he's back in the bathroom anyway, so I have a little time to hang out here and tell you about the magical events of my fifth year. But before I do, I would like to tell you about the few memories I have of another significant person in my preschool life.

Remember that I spoke briefly about my dad's father in the beginning? I really only have three memories of my paternal grandfather, or "Papa," as I called him. What's amazing to me is how dear these memories are to my heart. Some things in life you just can't explain, and that's all right.

The first memory of Papa was eating Chinese food at my parents' house with him, Nana, and my maternal grandparents. He radiated happiness. The second memory was at their house. I was playing on the floor. My brother yelled at me, "Go see Papa! He's very sick." So I went to see him, and they put me beside him in his bed. I just stayed close to him, without talking.

The final memory is sitting in my maternal grandparents' house, playing cards with my grandma and asking, "Where is everyone?"

"At Papa's funeral."

"What's a funeral?"

"They're putting Papa down for a very long nap."

"Okay. Go fish."

She did.

Those are my memories of Papa.

Meanwhile, Mac snuck into the kitchen and has begun to cook his traditional breakfast: vegetarian bacon, eggs scrambled hard, potatoes, whole wheat toast, and herb tea. Mac is a vegetarian, but not me! I gotta have an occasional White Castle hamburger or pepperoni pizza.

I really don't want to get out of bed this minute because my body aches with pain. I think I mentioned that before, however, I'm not sure if I did or not, because currently, my short term memory is blurred from all the damn pain! (Mac claims I always repeat myself and sometimes forget what I am saying, and maybe I do.) Anyway, it seems as if when I was younger, I was always in physical pain. And today is no different.

While Mac is taking his time preparing breakfast, all of a sudden the smells from the kitchen evoke a vivid recollection of my fifth year, sitting on the couch with my body cast, dying to go into the kitchen and get some homemade chocolate chip cookies. I couldn't move to save my life. I guess that's why I'm always on the run now, pain notwithstanding. I was actually an active kid despite my disability. But at the age of five, I did not realize how inactive I would soon become. I had to have a surgery to replace a hipbone. The surgeons took a bone from my foot and put it in my hip. It was a very painful recovery.

I can still visualize my hospital bed in detail and remember hearing my mom say in exasperation to my hospital roommate's mother, "They're little kids. Turn on *Sesame Street*, not the news!" I also remember my father complaining about the fact that he might not have a car to drive home because the hospital was in a rough part of the city. It's funny what kids remember. I'm sure he gave me a stuffed animal of Ernie because I was in love with that *Sesame Street* guy. I even ate with Ernie at every meal. He was the most dedicated guy I've ever met; next to Mac, of course.

When I came home from the hospital, my preschool class came over to make butter with me. It was kinda embarrassing having a bar across my legs and a cast up to my chest. I bet you're wondering how I did the necessary. Don't ask.

At the same time, believe it or not, my brother was envious of me. He broke his ankle and decided to keep me company in the old den. His company was okay, but he had control of the damn TV. He used to throw Goldfish crackers at me and laugh like a maniacal Woody Woodpecker. At least I had a normal childhood in that respect. My poor mother; all she heard was, "Mommy! Mommy!" Her unfailing reply was, "Steven, now cut that out!"

I was ecstatic when my parents said that I was getting my cast off. However, they did not tell me that I was going to still have to wear a brace at night, also with a damn bar between my legs. I distinctly remember the agonizing pain and screaming to my mom, "Take this off!" My sweet mommy, with her soothing voice, took the whole contraption off, and it felt so good. I guess it was a good thing that I couldn't take it off by myself.

I was also ecstatic to return to preschool because my dashing bus driver, Keith, picked me up for school every day. He was my heart's desire. Recently, I had a conversation with my mom, and I asked her, "How in the world did you realize that I had a crush on Keith?"

"Well, when your daughter jumps for joy when she sees the school bus, you know something is up." And, indeed, I had just started walking (and jumping) for the first time in my life after the brace and bar were permanently removed. I began to walk with my walker and coincidentally developed linguistic skills at the same time. Five years old was a milestone year.

I must add that I have had many, many operations over the years, and only that one at age five improved the quality of my life.

At the age of five and a half, I started kindergarten. I was delighted to show off my new skills and eagerly accompanied my mom to

Children's Specialized Hospital to meet Mrs. Stako. She informed my mom of a new school, Westlake School for orthopedically handicapped children in grades K through 8. Notice that I said, "orthopedically handicapped"; the lingo has changed so many times throughout my lifetime, I sometimes don't even know what to call myself! We found out that my kindergarten teacher would be a man. I remember going home and telling my brother Stevie that my kindergarten teacher was a boy. His name was Mr. Sandberg. My brother's reply was, "He might need some grass to put on his bald head." I really thought I needed grass to enter kindergarten. Happily, I found out that wasn't true.

Kindergarten was fun. Cindy and I were the two troublemakers. We were immensely curious about how Barbie dolls were made so what do you think we did? That's right; we took every Barbie completely apart. Mr. Sandberg couldn't understand why the Barbies were perpetually in pieces.

Besides the Barbies, a memory that stands out is when Mr. Sandberg gave us a math worksheet with a choo-choo train on it. I did all the math problems correctly and then had to color in the caboose. For example, the answer "four" represented the color green, three was yellow, and so on. I remember that doing the math was easy, but coloring was a pain. I implored, "I did my math, why do I have to color?" I finished well before everyone else, I had gotten a one hundred, and no way did I want to have to color in the lines of that damn caboose. And I knew my colors, too! Can you imagine a kid with absolutely no fine motor control whatsoever having to color prettily within the lines? No "reasonable accommodations" back then. Thanks, Mr. Sandberg, for being as unenlightened as the legislation. I guess he thought he was doing the right thing by me.

I returned home every day to my mom, who greeted me with celery sticks and raisins. I liked the raisins, I still do, but damn, where was I, in prison? Every other kid got cupcakes and cookies, and I got celery sticks. After my delicious snack, I went into the den and turned on *The Magic Garden*. I was content for about ten minutes until my brother came home from high school. Back then we had one television; imagine that. I think today's kids would freak out, don't you? He walked into the room and automatically turned off my *Magic Garden* to something stupid in its place, whatever that was. Sometimes we compromised and elected to watch Woody Woodpecker on channel five at three o'clock.

Up until the age of six, I was afraid of most things. I did not want Santa to come into my house because he might be a robber, who might even take my daddy. I was afraid of dogs, or anything that made loud, abrupt noises. The mother of one of my childhood best friends collected cuckoo clocks. They terrified me, and in order for me to go over to play, the girl's mom had to turn off fourteen cuckoo clocks. Today, we know why; however, back then no one understood the biological connection between CP and abrupt noises, sound sensitivity, light sensitivity, and the startle reflex. My fear reactions were mostly simple biology, not psychologically motivated. Mac and I will never have a dog because of my startle reflex.

At seven years old, I made my First Communion. Yes, I was Catholic back then. I recall being carried to church by my father. I remember my big party, in the new addition to our house. It was a beautiful den, overlooking the backyard that looked like park scenery with a pool. It was a terrific day. I got seven hundred and forty dollars in gifts, plus a watch, and I thought I could then move out with my three girlfriends, Jennifer, Lisa, and Kelly.

Obviously, some of my fears were diminishing, and even though I decided to stay at my parents' house for at least a few more years, I kept the friendship of those three girls. In fact, Kelly was my best friend for quite a while. She lived next door to me and was always over. Indeed, her father and my father were the best of friends and remain so today. Back then Kelly's daddy was going through a divorce with her mommy. Every Thursday night, while my mother was playing bridge, I was double dating with my dad and Kelly and her daddy. On Thursdays, we hit the town. I thought my daddy was the greatest, plus having my best friend by my side made everything ideal. When Kelly and her dad could not meet with us, I was a little upset because I had to share my dad with my sister, who would join us on those occasions. I was my daddy's girl, and I did not want to share him with anyone. All I cared about, besides those Thursday night daddy dates, were boys and trucks. You could say that I was a tomboy, but I was way too boy crazy to be a real tomboy.

When I came home from school after flirting with all my boyfriends, my mom had a tutor waiting for me. I don't know why because I was the smartest kid at school, plus, I thought my personality could win over anyone. My tutor's name was Diane. I think she talked to Gabrielle, my occupational therapist, about my charm because Diane did not fall for it. Diane brought me a book on multiplication and division and had me study it for weeks, even months.

"Why do I have to learn this when everybody else is still doing beginning addition; like one and one make two?"

"Because you are a very smart girl."

Like that made a lot of sense to me! If I was the smartest kid in my school, why did I have to do more homework than anyone else? One plus one does not equal two in this equation, does it? As a professor today, I ask my students what I mean by that, but you the reader are lucky enough to not have to do this assignment. So I will pretend to be a Ramapo student and explain it to you.

"Well, Professor Komoroski [soon to be Professor McCohnell], from a child's point of view, it is obvious why the little girl would be confused. But from the perspective of the concerned educator, it's clear that the child should be academically mainstreamed into a regular school, with nondisabled kids. However, back in your day —I am not saying that you're old, Professor K—the IDEA [*Individuals with Disabilities Education Act*] was not authorized until 1997. This was only 1982, and you were way ahead of your time."

I love when my students do the reading and use their analytical skills. Mac says that my students are my children. I want them to learn as much as they teach me. He also says that the students who irritate me the most teach me the most. True.

Ahhhh. I smell coffee, and he's calling me. Let's see what he wants. As I walk into the kitchen, not far from our bedroom, I feel better seeing coffee in my "Grumpy" mug. He greets me with a kiss and says, "Good morning again, Sleeping Beauty." But we all know that I'm not Beauty before my coffee, I'm Grumpy; who's he fooling?

As we eat breakfast, Mac is debating whether or not he should pick up extra work. As an in-demand respiratory therapist, he can usually work extra hours if he so chooses.

"Why are you gonna pick up work, if we're going out to dinner?"

"Exactly. That's my point. We need the money."

"Shit. We always need money. So what?"

That's right. If it were up to me, neither of us would have to work, and I would have my best buddy with me every day; I have always been a people person. But I know that we can always find a use for more money, even though we're financially comfortable. As a kid, I did my best to get out of physical therapy and speech therapy using my people skills. And now, with my future husband, I don't want him to go to work. I want him to stay home and play with me.

Speaking of playing, when my tutor left, I always had a half hour to go and play in my bedroom. On my ninth birthday, I received my own television. Archie and Edith Bunker always put me to sleep. I loved my little room next to mommy and daddy's room. And I loved my furniture because I had a big girl's bed, a TV with a remote, and a typewriter, on which I had to do my spelling words. I hated that typewriter; it was torture. To this day, I can neither spell nor type yet I don't think I'm doing too badly for myself.

All my girlfriends and I had sticker books, and I stored mine with pride in my room. My sticker book was the best. (If you talk to Jennifer, she would undoubtedly take issue with me.) As a child, I was very content in my bedroom, with the exception of the typewriter. I even had a goldfish that lived five years. I bet you're thinking, "How does a goldfish last five years?" I guess I was not very observant of my goldfish, for my pet had been replaced many times by my brother. Years later, when I was twenty-three, I learned that my brother had been feeding my goldfish to his snake, replacing my fish at least twenty times. Until then, I thought goldfish lived for five years.

As you can see, I was a happy kid with my little room, in between my parents and my sister. Those contented years waltzed serenely by.

One day at the age of ten, when I returned home from school, my mom was there with a decorator. I loved my room, but I haven't told you that my mother had to pick me up and put me in the tub to give me baths. The decorator was there to create my new room with an accessible bathroom and a walk-in shower. I was so happy. It was a joyful occasion, picking out all of the brand-new things for my new bedroom and new towels for my bathroom. The color was aquamarine. I even had a walk-in closet.

It's funny because while writing this, I suddenly realize that something major in my life happened every five years. Age ten was no exception. When my bedroom was completed, it was absolutely stunning. Out of nowhere, I blurted rebelliously to my mom, "I don't want it. I want my old bedroom." My mom said that was fine, knowing that eventually I would adjust. In fact, I did adjust very well to my new bedroom, sooner rather than later.

I didn't adjust to my sister Kim going away to college at Syracuse University. This period of my life was a sad, wobbly little section of my metaphorical staircase because my sister and I were very close and having her move out forever, to my youthful mind, was excruciating. She was about seven years older than me, and she had more of a maternal than a sisterly role in my life. The day was early in September 1984 when my parents and sister drove down the driveway, and I was left with the babysitter. I cried so hard, knowing that my sister was venturing into her new life, leaving me behind. My babysitter said to me that we should write Kim a letter that very day. Around six o'clock, the phone rang in my new room and I answered, "Hello?" It was my beloved sister.

Realizing that I had major loneliness in my heart, I was compelled to find meaningful substitutes in the likes of Jack Wagner and Jimmy Harding. Jack Wagner was "Frisco" on *General Hospital*, and Jimmy Harding was a boy in my school who had the worst acne ever, ever, ever, but he had my heart. I remember that he was the first boy who made my heart pound faster, and we secretly held hands when no one was looking. I would spend hours on the phone with him. He even gave me a silver chain and a love letter stating that I was his girlfriend. No one liked him because he was a wise-ass in school, but I happened to adore wise-asses. As you read on, you'll see this pattern continue in my life.

Nine months later, in the park, another classmate, Jose, pressured me to kiss Jimmy. I remember this as if it were yesterday. I kissed Jimmy with my eyes wide open! I was so nervous after the kiss that I immediately told Kelly I was pregnant.

"Oh my God! I think you should tell your mommy!"

It wasn't even a French kiss, and I thought I was pregnant. The image of *Love Boat* kissing scenes kept playing in my mind. On that show, casual kissing occurred a lot, and they did not use protection. After a day of worry, I disclosed to my mom that I was going to have a baby soon.

She knew I was not pregnant because at my age it was impossible, so her reply was, "How?"

"Well, you see, Mommy, I kissed Jimmy on the lips, and that's how I became pregnant." She then informed me a little about the birds and the bees, and my worries were diminished in a few minutes. Life was so simple back then and I went right back to kissing Jimmy, full tilt boogie.

During the course of my first love, I discovered my second love–Nassau in the Bahamas. Kelly, Kim, and I went to the Bahamas, and our parents were dragged along for the ride. I discovered what Paradise really was, and it was not New Jersey. The palm trees spoke to me, as did the beach and the azure waters, and I whispered to my daddy, "One day I am gonna live here with my husband." My dad just nodded his head and said, "That's nice, honey." Daddy didn't believe that this dream was reachable, but part of it will come true soon when I marry Mac, because we plan to honeymoon in the Bahamas. I believe that when we reach retirement, we'll make our final home in the Bahamas.

Back in preteen New Jersey, I was still Jimmy's girlfriend, and my young life continued to unfold.

The summer of 1986 was a memorable one indeed. My family rented a condo on Long Beach Island. I have come to realize in my life that family is not only biologically based. Family is based on how individuals interact with one another over a period of time, with the hope that the bond will remain close knit. The Stavitskis were a perfect example of family that was not biologically connected to me. "Aunt" Gina and my mom had decided that we should all go to Long Beach Island. Previously, we had stayed in comfortable suites at the Jersey shore in Wildwood Crest for the summer, but our fun in the sun vacation of 1986 was different. Both families shared a cramped, three-bedroom apartment, and that was the fun of it. Today if someone asked me what my favorite childhood vacation was, I would say those two weeks on Long Beach Island. Throughout my life, I have stayed at the best hotels and the worst hotels. Don't get me wrong, the five-star hotels are fabulous; however, the memories of good times with people we love can never be replaced with material opulence.

The memories of that summer include the raucous card games we started that actually lasted for years, until I was fifteen. My grandfather had taught me how to play poker for real money at the age of nine, and I was pretty damn good at the ripe old age of twelve.

Our apartment was right on the beach, accessible for everyone except me, because a walker and sand do not get along. The walker sinks into the sand and can't roll on the surface. My mom and Aunt Gina were very creative, using my snow sled to pull me over the sand dunes. I was then able to reach the glorious ocean without struggling. Luckily, I was a tiny kid, and my mom and Aunt Gina were very strong.

This was the summer before my adolescence, and Long Beach Island was the first place I experienced a social environment that showed me how different I was from my able-bodied peers. I loved the shore, but my sand-dune sled and non-swimming were markedly atypical. You'll see, as you continue to read, that my social life underwent many more dramatic changes in the next few years, but its genesis was that summer on Long Beach Island.

It was a hot, rainy afternoon. My sister was back at home, working for the summer. Aunt Gina's daughter Michelle was three years older than I was, and she had her girlfriend come down to visit, so there I was with my mom and aunt, all cozy and buddy-buddy, while my sister was at home, and my cousin had her best friend with her. Oh, I forgot to mention that my best friend, Kelly, was acting strange and weird and didn't want to come down to Long Beach Island with me.

My mom, Aunt Gina, and I were having lunch, discussing the topic of friends. I excused myself because I felt an urge to cry. I ran into the bedroom and slammed the door. My mom came into my tiny bedroom and asked me, "Christine, what's wrong? Why are you crying?"

"Mom, never mind. It's nothing."

"Why are you crying?"

Now, am I gonna tell her the truth? That I had no friends, and I was a big loser? And for the first time in my life, I hated my disability? Everyone was always telling me I was so special and so wonderful. If I was so damn special, why didn't I have any friends? I was obviously acutely different from my able-bodied peers.

"Mom, just forget it. You won't understand."

"Yes, I will, honey. I'm your mommy." And at that time, I believed her. At twelve years old, I still thought that my mommy could heal all my boo-boos. Come to think of it, till this day, I still think my mom can help heal a lot of my boo-boos.

"Mom, I don't have any friends, don't you see? I'm different. I'm not special. I'm just so . . . really, really different! I have no friends because I'm handicapped."

"That's not true, honey. You have lots of friends. You have Kelly, Jennifer, Michelle, your sister Kim, and your mother is always your best friend."

"I might be twelve, but I'm not stupid. Kelly and Jennifer haven't talked to me in a month. Michelle is Aunt Gina's daughter. Kim is my sister; she has no choice." I was also thinking, "God, am I really that much of a loser that my *mother* is my best friend?" Now that I'm a grown woman, I realize my closest friend *is* my mom. And I am pretty damn lucky. But back then I didn't want to hear that my mom was my best friend.

"Mom, you don't understand." I think I blamed her that I had a disability. I was so mean to her, but I was aware for the first time in my life of being trapped in an able-bodied society. This was a monumental and excruciating step in my very long staircase.

"I'm disabled because of you, Mom." Ouch.

In writing this, I realize that this was one of the most helpful things I ever said to my mom. Helpful, and revealing to both of us. I was a kid trapped. I was unaware of the pain that my parents were going through, and by blurting out that statement, I shared my feelings in a painful but galvanizing way.

My mom understood, and a couple months later she hired someone to take me out on the town once a week. Mom's idea was just perfect. My new companion and I went everywhere you can imagine in the world of energetic suburban adolescents, and it was all immensely appealing to me as an adventurous preteen. We had fun at the Jersey shore with all that yummy, healthy, boardwalk food like soft ice cream, cotton candy, fudge, pizza, hamburgers, French fries, corn dogs, onion rings, and so on. Aaah, those delicious smells and that ocean breeze. We also enjoyed good teen-movie comedies and the local restaurant where all the kids went. These outings provided a quick fix, enabling me to climb another step in my life's staircase. I used to think it was a short staircase but I was beginning to learn that it went on infinitely. Meanwhile, my Saturday nights out were a welcome relief.

In keeping with the fun social life with my new companion, just about everything else in life got much better, too. In seventh grade, I was elected Miss Westlake! *I was the most popular kid in my school.* Everybody adored me, even the teachers and the principal. I had it made. Mr. Hand, our bus driver, would pick me up at 7:20 in the morning. Then we would pick up Simmie, Allen, Kimberly (who was my best friend at Westlake), Alex, and Richard. We were inseparable, and we were the "cool group." On the ride to school, we would come up with a plan for the day. I was known to flirt with all the boys, but Jimmy still had my heart. Kimberly was the most subdued one and always told me to quiet down. Simmie was also quiet and sweet.

Richie and I were a pair and a half. He was in a wheelchair and had very little use of his arms due to spasticity. Allen and Richie went to the boys' room together so Allen could help Richie have a smoke. A thirteen-year-old today would probably laugh at this and say, "What's the big deal?" But back then it was a really big deal, especially in an all-orthopedically handicapped school. Of course, Allen and Richie came back smelling like smoke.

The next week, Miss Palmer taught the whole class, boys and girls together, all about the birds and the bees. Can you just imagine the conversation between us on the ride home? One adventurous boy said to me, "Do you want to have a baby, or try making one?"

"You're gross!"

Richie made comments about blood.

Kimberly said, "I would never have your baby if you were the last man on earth!"

The conversations about sex continued for a month. Little did I know that I would fall for that adventurous boy and one day say "yes" to his request.

Academically, I was doing well beyond my teachers' expectations. We were all hard workers, but I would completely finish my work by eleven o'clock every day and I began to get bored. Real bored. And when I get bored, I get into trouble. I still do today. Back then, I used to kiss the boys and talk too much to the teachers. My teacher, Mrs. Kimlicka, sent me to the principal's office every single day. In fact, the principal was very nice, but she didn't like talking to me every day.

My mom and dad asked me, "Why are you getting in trouble so much?"

"Who, me?"

They all realized that Westlake School was not the best setting for me to receive the best education. That June I graduated, and I was so excited. I didn't realize that one of the hardest years of my life was about to commence. Another giant step on the staircase of oppression.

Guess what? Mac has decided to run a couple errands. He is active, as you may have figured out, and he can't sit still for anything. But I must add that he does his zooming around with peace and tranquility.

I say to him, "Honey, why are you going out today?"

"Because I always have things to do on my days off."

"Like what?"

"Like the dry cleaners. Don't you like nice, clean clothes when you go to work? I'm your dry cleaner man."

"Oh, that's right, honey. My suit *is* at the cleaners."

"And, honey, you need it for Saturday night. Besides, you get all nervous before you go to work. I'm gonna leave so you can go through your routine pre-class jitters."

He has a point there. I always run around the house like a damn chicken with its head cut off before I leave for campus. I often forget that *I'm* the professor, and I have little reason to be nervous. I think it just means that I simply desire to teach the students to the very best of my capabilities.

As he gets up from the table, Mac kisses me and says, "Good-bye, Lucy." That's his nickname for me because I'm often absent-minded, just like the old *I Love Lucy* TV show. "I'll see you at the Thai restaurant at about 9:30 tonight."

"Does that mean you're not picking up extra work tonight?"

"You're the professor. Figure it out. Love you."

I hear him say as he's leaving, "Good morning, Edwina."

"Good morning, Mac."

The staircase of my life is stable and steady this morning.

I sit daydreaming at the kitchen table, watching the cars go by.

My Teenage Years and Young Adulthood

"Good morning, Christine."

"Good morning, Mamita. How are you today?"

Edwina walks into the kitchen, takes off her jacket, and sits down at the kitchen table. I think society puts too damn much emphasis on defining people by their occupations rather than taking an integrated look at who they are as a person. Edwina is occupationally defined as my housekeeper; however, she is more like a friend. If anyone has seen the movie *Crash,* which I show to my First Year Seminar class at Ramapo, I relate to Sandra Bullock's character because her housekeeper was her friend, and in times of need, the housekeeper was the only one there for her character. That's the way I sometimes feel about Edwina.

As we have our usual pleasant morning conversation, ten minutes have passed.

"Oh my God, Edwina! I gotta go to work!"

"Yes, Mamita. You better get going soon!"

I "hop" into my accessible walk-in shower, and Edwina is in my closet picking out something for me to wear to work. Even today, I cannot pick out clothes for the life of me, so I have a personal shopper who buys my clothes—good ol' Mom. I will call my mom and inform her that I need new clothes. The next week, she comes over with clothes and the bill. I write out the check for the bill and give her some extra for her services. This method works wonders, but I always try to be creative in my outfits, and Edwina always rejects them. I have no time to be creative *and* argue with Edwina. Today clothes do not have a big impact on my success. Hell, I don't even dress myself anymore, but back in the summer of 1987, things were totally different.

It was July 11and I got a huge gift–a brand new scooter was delivered to me. I was so excited, and I had two glorious months to practice on my electric scooter before starting at my new school. My sister had some friends over, and I remember feeling so cool driving my black scooter–so cool that I drove right into the bushes.

"Help! Help!"

"Christine, what are you doing?"

"What do you think? What does it look like I am doing?" I was clearly stuck in the bushes, and people were asking something foolish like what I was doing?!

My mother bellowed from the house "Don't drive so fast!"

At that point, I began to comprehend that my reality was going to be different not just from society at large, but from that of my family members, as well. They were able-bodied and not scooter users, among many other differences. And even though I sensed a new world ahead, I didn't comprehend the impact its changes would bring to the next six months of my life.

September 1987 marked my entry into Hillside Avenue School in Cranford, New Jersey. It was the only junior high school in Union County that was accessible back in those days. Even though the legal regulations had been passed in 1977 enacting the federal accessibility law known as 504 (remember?), accessibility in public schools was not enforced. Anyway, Hillside Avenue School was architecturally accessible, but I was the only physically disabled student enrolled. Damn! Just guess how that made me feel.

My first vivid memory of seventh grade (which this "A" student had to repeat simply to be admitted to the school) was having a conversation with Miss Peters. She was explaining how, at that school, students switched classes, and the teachers would let me out a few minutes early so it would be easier for me to get to my next class.

As the weeks went on, it dawned on me that I was not making any friends. I also began to realize that the work was much too easy for me. I forgot to mention that I was in all Resource Room classes. These were classes primarily for students with learning, developmental, and intellectual disabilities. The school officials and educators assumed that because I had CP, I must have a low IQ and no problem-solving skills. I'm not implying anything negative about our brothers and sisters who have intellectual disabilities, but it has always unnerved me to have folks not recognize my fairly obvious intelligence. (At least, in my opinion, it's obvious!) The students in my classes were all cognitively disabled, and, in my thirteen-year-old opinion, all geeks. Well, I was smart, smart-alecky, and no geek! In due course, the school decided to put me in "regular" math and English classes, where I excelled. Nevertheless, I soon cried to Miss Peters that even though the schoolwork was more at my level, I still had no friends.

"I know a really nice girl that you can eat lunch with."

I was so excited. I came to find out that she was the biggest geek in the whole school! I was mortified. Here I was, the coolest kid on the block last year, and this year I was eating with the biggest geek in school. Then I realized that everyone was picking on me. I didn't understand why. Back then, I could dress cool and I knew I looked cool. I just knew it. So what was wrong?

A girl named Charlene really had it in for me. "I'm gonna beat you up, retard!"

What could I have said? "No, I'm gonna beat *you* up, asshole!" I knew I didn't have a chance. I didn't know why everyone was so freakin' mean to me. That can be hard on a kid. I started to develop panic attacks as a result of my fears of school. It was then that I realized having a disability really, really sucked. In a couple of weeks, my innocence had been taken away. Robbed innocence, social exclusion, and discrimination by my peers became permanent in my daily life. More steps on the damn staircase.

My days of sibling rivalry with Stevie about the television were over, now replaced by truly dismal tears and misery. I couldn't understand why I was not cool at my new school because every Friday night, I would hang out at the local church with my old friends who all had disabilities. With them I was totally, undeniably cool.

"Christine, there's a ghost in the other room, and he wants to have sex with you."

"F--- you."

But on Monday, I turned into a timid geek. Did I sound like a geek to you? Just think how confused I was.

My brother's friend, Lenny, talked to me after school. We were eleven years apart, but I had a crush on him. He was always telling me, "Christine, when you get older, kids won't be as mean." I was thinking, "Just kiss me, Lenny," but later in the evening, I wondered what he meant. I was pissed off that he had not resolved the problem at that moment—both the meanness of the kids *and* the kissing. What was I to do? My sister was away at college and this time, I literally had no friends. Of course, I still had my friends from Westlake, but I thought I was too good for them at this stage. Little did I know you're never too good for anybody.

I began to wonder what life meant, and my panic attacks continued. Why couldn't I just be happy, like a normal kid? Why me? What is my purpose? Why are people mean to each other? At the age of thirteen, one should not be concerned with these existential "adult" issues. So what did my parents do? They took me to see a good ol' shrink.

My mom and I entered the shrink's office. I was a quiet, shy, timid teenager; yes, I was shy at that one sad point in my life. After several sessions with the shrink, she diagnosed me as having panic attacks. She put me on Prozac. "Shit," I thought. "I'm really messed up. Now I'm on meds." After that I seemed okay, at least on the outside. In our therapy sessions, the shrink didn't make a lot of sense to the thirteen-year-old me.

I remember her saying, "Christine, you are a very intelligent little girl, and the compulsiveness of your thinking illustrates that you are very mature." For me, that didn't mean anything. My compulsive nature and maturity were related? Pretty soon, I realized that she had her own agenda. Okay, just give me my happy pills, and let me go on my merry way. In fact, the pills did help me to not worry about every damn thing and allowed me to think about more important things, like being cool.

In the beginning of eighth grade, things changed drastically. During that summer, I had many conversations with myself, as I became aware of my growing up. I also started thinking about my own values and beliefs. These self-conversations coincided with events on the first day of eighth grade. I was placed in three mainstream classes, and my other classes that were in the Resource Room had all the really *bad* kids in it. I was in heaven! Listen up, it gets better: My aide was Mrs. Mark; she was the coolest woman in the school! She made me laugh so much during class that *both* of us got kicked out. It was then that I discovered I had a sense of humor and started to surround myself with a whole bunch of friends, who enjoyed my style of smart-ass comic relief. The odd thing was that I was bad as hell, but the teachers loved me because I was a smart, *academic* role model. Sometimes having CP and smarts really paid off.

There are so many good memories of eighth grade. As I sit here reminiscing, I would like to share just a few with you. Oh, by the way, I was fifteen. Remember what I said about my every-five-years milestones? At this joyful point, the staircase of my life was breezy and accessible. Any way you look at it, I was one happy, spunky girl.

"Will you kids pay attention in the kitchen?!" yelled Miss Warner at us four unruly students in cooking class. Trish, Jeremy, Brian, and me. We were the very bad kitchen group in the class. Trisha was the mother hen of the misfits. Brian was the Swedish Chef from the Muppets, always talking in that silly gibberish. Jeremy, the pothead, was always burning himself when he fell asleep by the stove. And there I was, cracking up at them and trying to cut pieces of celery with the deft, fine motor skills of CP. That was quite a kitchen. We had so much fun that we didn't care if we got an A or an F. I think we got Ds. Who would have thought that this misfit group would produce a nurse, a cop, a dad of two, and a professor? I'm sure Miss Warner would need to see documentation to believe it. Trish and I still remain friends. And guess what? My first official date was with Jeremy—the pothead!

We met at a movie theater in Westfield, New Jersey. The scent of his cologne is still very much in my mind. We saw *The Freshman*. Well, in truth, we didn't actually *see* the movie because what happens in the back row of movie theaters never changes. Get my drift? If you don't, ask your parents. I'm sure they did the same thing we were doing.

Excuse me; I'm forced to digress. As I get dressed this morning, my body is fussy and achy, and I wonder why God has given me the body I have, with spasms and involuntary movements that make my life arduous. However, as I'm talking to you, I realize that my life today is as "normal" as anyone else's, maybe even better. I am a soon-to-be wife. I have a college education. I am a professor of Disability Studies. I'm a taxpayer, a voter, and I'm trying to compromise with my mom on plans for my wedding album.

My life in eighth grade was in tandem with that of my nondisabled peers. Mrs. Mark had a unique place in my life because while she was my aide in school, assisting me with my academic work, she really enhanced my social arena. Even though my academic work was important, and I excelled, Mrs. Mark taught me so much more. She adapted herself to fit in with my "bad" friends.

What I remember most about eighth grade was holding in my laughter on a daily basis, and that was a pretty difficult task, taking into consideration that involuntary CP movement always accompanied my laughter. Major spasticity and laughter. What a sight I was! Can you just picture it? "Christine, if you do not stop laughing, I will have to kick you out!" thundered the science teacher.

My reputation of being a bit of a devil was growing. I had it all. And every time I have it all (like getting good grades and having an active social life), I get interrupted due to circumstances surrounding my disability.

"Christine, what's your schedule for next year? Do you have math second period? Maybe we have the same math class."

"What the hell are you talking about, Trisha?"

"Didn't you get your schedule for next year?"

"No."

Know why I didn't get my schedule for next year? Because I was going to a different school. Why? Because the neighborhood high school was not accessible. It was 1989, the year before *The Americans with Disabilities Act*. Technically, as I've already stated, *The Rehabilitation Act* of the 1970s had provided the legislation for all government buildings (like public schools) to be fully accessible to people with disabilities, but as I have *also* already stated, the law was not enforced. I had no choice but to go to a different, accessible school, starting all over again. Shit.

The summer between eighth and ninth grade, I found myself again contemplating why my life was so difficult. Luckily, entering

David Brearley High School in Kenilworth, New Jersey, wasn't quite as traumatic as entering junior high school, due to the familiar faces I remembered from Westlake. The reason why I saw so many familiar faces was because in New Jersey, there was only one accessible high school per county in the early 1990s. As a result, every teenager who had a physical disability in my county went to my new high school. Great! I knew all of 'em!

Automatically, I thought it would be like old times, but two years is like a lifetime when you're an adolescent. David Brearley was a public school, and it had only one self-contained class for all physically disabled students, grades nine through twelve. As well as attending the self-contained class, some of the kids were mainstreamed. Fortunately, I was one of them. Maybe that would help widen my social life, which was always a top priority to me.

The summer before my freshman year of high school was an adventure. I had my friends in Cranford and my friends at Westlake. One day that eventful summer, I was talking to my friend Kimberly. Remember her? She was crazy about this boy named Fred. But Fred was a little full of himself—okay, a lot full of himself. He didn't like Kimberly.

She called me while I was playing Milli Vanilli and Bob Marley (not at the same time!). I had certainly gotten used to my new room by then. The music was blasting, and my phone almost never stopped ringing.

"Kim, what's wrong?"

"Fred doesn't want to talk to me any more on the phone."

"Oh, yeah? Give me his phone number, I'll call him."

"No, no, no!"

"Okay. But I think he's on our bus, and I'll talk to him."

"No, please—well, okay."

And I was right; he *was* on the bus.

The first day of high school on that bus was very interesting. I was the first one on at 7:20 in the morning. Then we picked up some kid—I don't even remember his name. The next stop was Fred. I recall it all so clearly. I thought to myself, "Fred, my ass." As he came out of his house, he walked funny, and he wasn't even cute. He was dark, darker than dark. He walked on the bus and started talking to the other kid.

29

"Yo, man, Kim calls me all the time, and I never return her phone calls. She's a pain in my ass."

Right then, I wanted to unbuckle my seatbelt and beat the shit out of him. Then I realized he was a boy, and I was a girl. So, I sat back and observed everything. Next stop was Kimberly. She got on the bus, introduced us, and all hell broke loose! Our bus driver wasn't interested in our loud volleys. All she said was, "I hear language from you kids that I don't even hear from my husband!" Our arguments lasted for at least two weeks. Then I realized Fred wasn't a bad guy, after all. Kim just really annoyed him.

Today Fred is one of my dearest friends. He's someone on whom I can count for anything and everything. We had a love affair on and off for five years, from the time I was seventeen until I was twenty-three. Actually, I was never in love with him, but we had a real, true bond, and we still do.

But back then we were two kids from opposite sides of the tracks. I was an "upper class" white girl, and he was African American and "ghetto cool." We complemented each other so well that we were inseparable. Kinda like Stanley and Ollie, sometimes even like Superman and Lois. Always together.

One day, I got on the bus, crying.

"Fred! They always pick on me. John C. called me a retard, and Donald J. called me stupid. And I have no friends in this school," I complained, not realizing that one of the greatest friends of my life was sitting right in front of me.

"Don't you worry. I'll take care of you."

Thinking to myself I wondered, "How's he gonna take care of this?"

The next day, John C. and Donald J. were so nice to me at lunch that I questioned my girlfriend, "What is going on?"

"You didn't hear? Louon chased John and Donald down the hall and scared the shit out of them." Fred was best friends with the enormous football captain, Louon. From that day forward, I had no problem with friends at Brearley. No one ever bothered me after that. In fact, John and I became friends.

My life at high school sailed on. I can never forget my first high school crush. His name was Jit. The third marking period, I had adaptive gym (a class adapted to students with disabilities) by myself. Later on, Jit joined me because he had broken his ankle. I was so in love with him. He was the ultimate Guido, and I loved the smell of his cologne. It was cheap and wonderful. We had gym five days a week for forty-five minutes each class. That was a lot of time together.

"I think I'm falling in love!"

"Oh, I see you have friends now, and you're even falling in love," replied Fred.

Those bus conversations were priceless. I learned more outstanding details concerning the birds and the bees; I learned what "hot" meant— not weather hot. Not looking hot either. Not boyfriend hot. Get my drift? Let me explain.

Fred got on the bus one day with a really cool boom box. Yes, in those days we did not have MP3 players or iPods. The bigger the boom box, the better it was. Fred sat down and put his big boom box right next to us. Five minutes went by.

"Fred, that's a nice boom box."

"Yeah, it's hot."

"Well, put it in the shade on the seat in front of you, so the sun won't blast it."

You can see the cultural differences between Fred and me were quite distinct, but the bond between us couldn't have been stronger. He never told me from whom he had stolen the magnificent boom box.

A lot of people in high school assumed that I was a snob, and now that I look back, I was to some extent. But not *totally* a snob, just a teenager from a family that had quite a bit of money. Sandy Barabosa thought that I was the biggest snob going. And I thought that she was the biggest nerd around. We didn't get along at all. As time progressed, we became good friends, but Trisha was still my best, best girlfriend back then. We were inseparable. She even went with my family and me on one of our many Club Med vacations, where "Tipsy" Chris always won the award for being the wildest. Yes, I was "Tipsy" and consumed a lot of alcohol (procured by my brother Stevie) on those fun vacations. Stevie and I would always dance at the disco. Then in the morning, other vacationers would come up to me and express how wonderfully I could party and dance. It felt so damn good to feel free on the dance floor. I felt so empowered and proud of my dancing technique. In fact, years later in 2000, I resumed dancing with a semi-professional dance troupe.

In January of 1990, my brother Charlie and his then-fiancée asked me to be in their wedding on September 9. I was so happy. Traci had a good heart. Along with the news of Charlie being engaged, another exciting thing was occurring. My *truly* best, best, best friend was coming home from college–my sister Kimberly! I was absolutely thrilled to have her home. My mom had a surprise graduation party for her, and Trisha and I got a little tipsy there, too. Life was good back then.

On March 9, 1990, my mom and dad threw *me* a big Sweet Sixteen party. It was at our favorite restaurant in Fanwood, New Jersey, Rodolpho's. There were about one hundred guests. We had a DJ, we had a cartoonist, and guess what? Jeremy the Pothead was my date! Trisha came. Kimberly from Westlake came, too, and Fred was her date. (By the next year, *I* was dating Fred.) I remember my maternal grandma sitting at my party, looking stunningly beautiful. My maternal grandfather and I danced. God, I miss them both. I also miss my dear paternal grandparents, as I've said. I think about all of them every single Sunday and wonder if they would be proud of who I am today. I just wish they could come back for one day—to my wedding. I miss them so much that it hurts. But back to the party. The pothead and I danced the night away. Picture this: Me on my walker jumpin' and jivin', and Jeremy intermittently taking both my hands so I could boogie without the walker. I'm sure all the men in my family, especially Stevie, were watching every move he made. I still hold fond memories of that day because I can look at the photographs in my Sweet Sixteen album.

During the summer of 1990, I shocked my parents to death. Oh, they're still alive, but the shock *could* have killed them.

"Mom!"

"Yes, Christine, what's the matter?"

"Can we talk?"

"Uh-oh, every time you say that, you're up to something."

"I just wanna talk to you. I have to learn how to drive. I just have to!"

"*What?* I don't know, Christine. We have to talk to your father about this one."

Oh, damn, I must have really said something because she rarely says that to me. Later, at dinner, I discussed the matter with my father. I felt as if I were twelve, when I had tentatively broken the extremely important news to him that I had become "a woman." As it turned out, then and now, I didn't need to be wary of my dad's reaction because he was always happy about progress in my life. Of course, he was glad about my spunky attitude about driving. That's my dad. Anyway, doesn't every sixteen-year-old kid want their driver's license?

Two weeks later, my mom told me that she had enrolled me in a special driving school for people with disabilities. I was so excited!

"Oh my God, Mom, thank you so much!"

Two weeks after that, I went for my first lesson. I didn't like the instructor, and he didn't like me. Following an hour on the road, he asked me to come into his office. I knew this wasn't a good sign. He sat my mother and me down and told us in his fancy mumbo jumbo that I was unable to drive. I was devastated beyond belief, and I cried all that night. I felt that my independence was taken from me; my normalcy was robbed. I was the oldest of all my friends who still couldn't drive. I really felt like shit, and again I hated my disability.

"My parents should have put me in an institution. Dammit. I'd be better off," I thought to my teenage self melodramatically. The desire to be "normal," everything around me; it all sucked. My social success on the rickety stairway to heaven seemed impossible to reach with this new obstacle.

Oops! Back to present day.

"Mamita, Mamita! Do you need this?"

"Yes, Mamita," I reply hurriedly. "Thank you so much."

Without Edwina helping to keep me organized, I would never leave this house. Remember, Mac calls me "Lucy," and for good reason. I can be extraordinarily absent minded, even though I'm a hard-working professor. Disorganized, absent minded, intelligent, detail oriented, forgetful, passionate—all in one person.

"Shit!" I always curse at my garage. It's too damn small for this van. Shit again! Now I did it; there's another big scratch on the door. Mac is gonna be very unhappy about a new scratch.

I'm meeting my dear friend and boss, Mike Fluhr, in the office, and I'm driving real fast to Ramapo College. (I'm not making up the fact that we are genuine friends. I'm sure you've noticed that I talk a lot about friends and how vital they are to me. I'm fortunate to have experienced so many friendships in my life.) Okay, okay, back to my speeding along the highway to meet him.

"Do I have time to stop for an iced latte?" I ask myself. "Mike isn't always on time anyway, and five minutes won't make a difference. Will it?" I pull into a van-accessible parking spot, lower my ramp, hop on my scooter, and whisk off to Starbucks. Sometimes I'm lucky, and someone can hold the door for me. Starbucks is one of the most accessible coffee houses in 2006, but their doors are far too heavy for people with disabilities to open, which is common with "accessible" doors everywhere. I'm in luck today, and someone is holding the door.

"Thank you."

"No problem."

I scoot in.

"Hi, Christine. The usual?"

"Yes, my usual. Thanks, Carrie. Iced vanilla latte, light on the ice. Thanks, Jim. Have a good day." Oh, shit, now I'm *ten* minutes late! I may talk slow and walk slow, but I drive mighty fast. Pedal to the metal, baby, that's me! And the left lane down 287 is lots of fun. When I'm behind the wheel, that's the only time I feel positively equal to everyone else. Maybe unconsciously, it's where I get my frustrations out. Imagine if I hadn't kept my driving lessons a secret from my parents at the age of seventeen, and hadn't learned how to drive–I don't even want to think about where my frustration would have led me.

I haven't told you the second half of my driver's license story, but now's the perfect time, as I'm speeding along 287.

The day after receiving the devastating news that I could not attain a driver's license, I went to school crying. I had adaptive gym by myself that day.

"What's the matter, Chris? What do you have to be upset about, Miss Troublemaker Herself?" asked Jim, the gym teacher.

"Jim, I can't drive. This sucks. This really sucks."

"What do you mean, you can't drive? I saw you drive. You drive well."

You see, a week earlier, Jim had taken me out in this old car that was used for Driver's Ed. He said he could teach me, but my parents then changed their minds and decided that they wanted the best driving instructor for adolescents with disabilities. The most expensive, I have learned, does not necessarily mean the best. I think a lot of people have that misconception.

"I'll teach you how to drive, Chris."

"You will? But only one stipulation," I said. "Don't tell my parents." I didn't want them to have a heart attack.

Off we went, Jim and me, on the road. This little Buick, about twelve years old, happened to have a "suicide knob," which allowed me full rotation on the steering wheel with one hand. And a left-foot accelerator. Like I said, off we went!

"Mom, could you pick me up from school around five o'clock tomorrow?"

"Why?"

Damn. What am I gonna say? I know. "I'm doing a group project, and we need time in the library." Yeah, that's a good one! Would she believe it? She never caught on that I had quite a few group projects after school that marking period. While she thought I was in the library, I was really on the Garden State Parkway or the New Jersey Turnpike or Route 22, or some other roads that were not too safe. I apologize to any non-New Jersey readers for my reference to local landmarks, but those days were fun.

The big day for my license test came in April. I remember going to Plainfield to the DMV. I took my test and asked the instructor, "I failed, didn't I?"

He said to me, "Do you want to fail?" Silence. "Congratulations, Christine. You got your driver's license."

I was overjoyed, and then I thought, "How am I ever going to tell my parents?" I just went home and timidly told my mom, shaking in my shoes.

"Mom, I got my license."

"The license for your scooter?"

"No, my driver's license."

"We'll talk to your father at dinner. Go to your room and do your homework."

Why am I always sent to my room, and later I have to divulge my story to my family at the dinner table? Maybe that's why to this day I don't like eating there. At the dinner table, I was shaking in my shoes again. My mom said to me slyly, "Why don't you tell your father the great news?" I knew full well she did not mean "great news" in any genuine sense.

I told him very, very quickly and tried my utmost to slur my words.

To my great surprise and delight, my daddy was happy for me.

"Whew!" I exhaled to myself. "Thank God."

His response was that I should never let anyone tell me what I could or couldn't do in life. I felt like all the barriers to freedom had been lifted from me at long last. Boy, was I dead wrong.

Damn! Why are so many other drivers on 287 North always on my ass? I'm going 80! Dammit! I'm zooming along in my super-nifty accessible silver van with its retractable ramp and my electric scooter, plus my extra walker, in the back. I have a left-foot accelerator and a spinner knob, the one I called a suicide knob as a teenager.

Back then I remember asking, "Mom, why do I have to take off a day from school because Drive-Master wants to take my measurements?" (Drive-Master is a company that modifies vehicles for disabled drivers.)

"Okay, never mind, you can go to school. We'll pick you up afterwards, but Christine, why are you so mad at everyone these days?"

She did not realize that I just wanted my van and my freedom. Drive-Master had already taken my measurements for the van and lost them. I was understandably impatient by now. A nondisabled kid can just hop into their parents' car and drive. I was unable to do that because, of course, my vehicle needed accessibility accommodations. I was beginning to feel resentment toward my disability once again.

So, my parents came to pick me up from school, and my sister was with them. I didn't catch on because other things were on my mind, as we drove to Drive-Master. I simply thought we were all together so that we could go out to dinner afterward. A worker there asked me to get into a van so they could measure me once again. My response was not so cooperative, but because my dad gave me a disgruntled, commanding look, I had no choice but to play along. I got in the van and soon noticed that everything I needed was already in there. The salesman asked me how I liked *my* brand-new van, and I was ecstatic, but I also felt bad because I had just been so rude to that nice man.

My mom drove the van home because I was too chicken. My mom's parents were waiting there, and we all celebrated. My grandfather turned to me and said, "See, this time, I'm the only one who believed in you." We know that's not true because without my gym teacher, I would never have had the golden opportunity of the driving lessons in that old car at David Brearley School. And *I* had believed in myself.

My grandfather then gave me a very important card and maybe it's why I drive too damn fast. He was a former police officer, so Grandpa provided me with a PCA card. That's a card that you get when you support the police union. Basically, it saves your ass if you are speeding on 287, as Professor McCohnell (my soon-to-be married name!) does, on a regular basis.

"Here you go, Chris," said my grandfather.

"What's this for?"

"Don't worry, Chris, you'll know it when you need it. Come on, take me for a ride."

Do you have a memory or two that you recall so clearly you can remember the scent of that particular time and place? For me, this was such an occasion.

I got into my brand-spanking-new van. My father sat in front, my grandfather got into the back because he claimed that he wanted to be chauffeured to Sears on Route 22 (about a ten-minute ride from my parents' house). When we returned, he said he had never been so scared in his life and he never let me forget it—even in my very last conversation with him.

I thought I had it made. My driver's license, my own vehicle, and off I went. Boy, how wrong I was. As a teenager, you tend to think you know it all, and I was no exception. I thought I was hot shit. As usual, Mom had a much different point of view.

I tend to forget that my life is markedly different from the vast majority of nondisabled folks. I forget that the internal, unconscious level of chaos I experience is not typical. It's not as ominous as that last statement sounds. It's just that my wild, free spirit is always ready to rumble, ready for the next stupendous adventure, like getting my driver's license. You'll hear this from me many times. It's my mantra. That is the exact opposite of how most people view someone with a disability, especially a young female.

Anyway, back to my mom's different point of view. New Jersey law did not require a teenage driver with a disability to have a licensed adult driver in the car, so I was indeed ready to rumble, but Mom insisted that either she or Dad had to be in the car whenever I drove. Alas, so much for my driving to wild parties, which is just where I wanted to go!

That night, I grabbed my keys (just like my older siblings always had). "Mom, Dad, I'm going to Trisha's. Be back later."

"What? No, you're not! Are you crazy?"

You can just imagine the "conversation" that followed. But I sincerely didn't understand my mother's point. We often hear "I'm living with the teenager from Hell." And that same teenager says in return, "My parents are such assholes." But do we ever stop to analyze the confusion of both parties? Hell, I didn't at that time, either. I think that was the first time my mom and I had a mother-daughter fight. My recollection is that we didn't care about the other's perspective. We just wanted what we wanted. Of course, I wanted my freedom, and Mom was prolonging my childhood. We had many disagreements during the summer of 1991. The ironic part is I honestly don't remember when she finally let me go out on my own. To this day, I dread driving my mother anywhere. I dread the day when she can't drive, and I'll have to play chauffeur. I bet my mother dreads the same thing. I can predict the telephone call thirty years from now: "Mac, can you please take your mother-in-law to the store? Please?"

Fred and I started to date in October 1991. You know how people have regrets in their life? Well, this is one of the biggest regrets I've ever had. I was never in love with him; I led him on for five years. Maybe I've just forgotten the intensity that we had. I never told my parents about him because he was African American, and I was afraid of what their reaction to him would be. I once tried to tell my mom about Fred, and she said that she would never accept it, that I couldn't date him. So I lived a dual life for no legitimate reason at all. I did this for eleven years—until I met my husband. I was in therapy during the initial stages of this part of my life. At that time I realize the benefit therapy could have been to me, and didn't feel that it was a help.

There was excitement to having a dual life. The constant sneaking around took a lot of brainwork. It made sense to me. In sports, you can win a game. It was the same idea here. Getting away with something, adding drama to one's life, how thrilling is that? Mischief has always intrigued me.

It amazes me because I was not doing anything wrong by dating an African American man. I'm married to one now. (Obviously, I'm writing my memoir in real time, and Mac and I have married.) But back then, I felt so wrong for dating on the sly and going against my parents. I didn't realize that I was right this time, and they would eventually change their views. Maybe I thought he was the only man I would "get." Now that I'm writing this, I think *How racist was I? I was the biggest racist of them all.* It's so painful that I can hardly write about it. I lied to my parents for years. I made up an imaginary friend named Joanne (aka Fred). Dating and my parents never mixed. The following paragraphs will give you some insight to my personal relationships. Please excuse my lack of chronology, but my brain seems to take time lines and intertwine them to make up a tapestry that ultimately makes sense to me.

By now, I'm sure you realize that I was boy crazy. When I was "dating" Fred, it was magical: my first "true love." I had a minivan, too.. It was a whole different world when I was with him. Often I melodramatically considered killing myself because I couldn't bear to tell my parents, and I couldn't bear to break up with Fred. From seventeen to nineteen we were together, and then we were on again, off again for the next several years. My early dating years were deliciously clandestine…and rocky.

I also had a crush on a guy, Dan Fusco. Boy, he was hot! But he never liked me, and I knew why–because of my rotten disability. Maybe that's why I stuck with Fred. Fortunately, as time went on, I became a proud woman with a disability and no longer saw my CP as a rotten handicap.

Fred and I first broke up right before my entering Ramapo College. I was devastated. I mourned, "Oh, my God! My whole world is gonna

end!" He said we should date other people, and I said, "F--- you."
Strangely enough, I wanted to date other people, too. Go figure.

The first semester at Ramapo College was the best and the worst
semester of my life. I moved into my dorm room. My friend Barbara
had been taking summer classes and working, and she knew of some
guy in a wheelchair who wanted to hang out with us. I shrugged, "Okay,
I'll go."

"He's in an apartment, and we can drink all night."

"Now you're talkin'. Let's get drunk and high at the same time,
girlfriend." (Good joke! Isn't that what all college kids said?)

We went to his apartment, and I thought they made a cute couple
together, Barbara and Ken. But as the weeks went on, he kept pursuing
me. And I kept watching him drum with his wondrous feet in the music
studio, where he was also an incredible rap artist. Even now, I get chills
thinking about it. We connected, or at least I thought we did. I'm sure
he had other things on his mind. I fell in love with him, and I later lost
my virginity to him—with my avid consent.

Taking a break from rapping and drawing with his feet, Ken had a
very seductive way about him. His soft, tender kisses made me believe
that he was *the one*. I remember the night: It was getting late, and we
were both studying for midterms.

He said, "Go back to the dorm room. Get some rest because I'm
gonna give you a night that you'll remember for the rest of your life."
And boy, was he right!

At midnight (for college students that's the middle of the day), I
heard a knock on my door. But it was quite different from a regular
knock because he knocked with his feet, not his hands. I opened the
door.

In the early nineties, we only had cassette tape players. No iPods,
no MP3s, and no CD players. R&B was playing and setting the mood.
One thing led to another in my tiny twin bed. The dorm room was
small too, so my scooter and his electric wheelchair were a tight fit.

This is going to show my age, but I remember very clearly the
setup of the Brady Bunch house. Three boys in one room; three girls
in another room; a bathroom connecting them. My dorm room had
a similar setup but with two people in one room sharing a bathroom
with the other two-person bedroom. While Ken and I were busy,

my hip went out. I screamed, but fortunately the jab of pain went away quickly. Unfortunately, Denise, a young woman from across the hallway, who is today one of my treasured friends, heard my scream and was understandably concerned. She ran to my room, but the door was locked. So she ran into my suite-mate's room, dashed through the bathroom, and still has nightmares about what she had seen. That poor, shocked eighteen-year-old freshman girl flew out of the room, yelling to anyone and everyone what she had just inadvertently witnessed.

Of course, the next morning, everyone knew that Ken and I had made love.

"I thought you wanted to keep this on the DL," accused Fred.

I replied, "I'm in love!" (On that magical night, Ken had also dedicated a song to me: "Adore" by Prince.)

The love affair went on for a couple of months. Well, actually, it was couple of weeks. Yes, I lost my virginity to a player—a helluva sexy one, though.

During Thanksgiving break, we went our separate ways. He called me the first week of break, and I did the same. The second and third day, he never responded to my phone messages. I was pissed off. When we returned to school, he kept avoiding me and did not show up at my dorm room. He was performing at a Step Show and claimed that he was too busy. He came over just once, and we made passionate love once again.

His roommate and I were publicizing the Step Show event. The night of the show, Ken was still claiming that he was practicing diligently, but he also mentioned that he had "clicked" with a woman back home. My wary response was, "What the hell does that mean?"

"I don't know yet."

"Well, I'll see you at the show."

I was sitting with all the key people on the lowest bleachers in the gym and wondering where Ken was. All of a sudden, I saw him walk in with a woman on his arm. With her, he was ambulatory, as well. Needless to say, I went ballistic! My friend Denise and her date, as well as everybody at the event, could not believe how absolutely out of control I became. I think I could have handled it a little better if Ken had not sat her directly behind me and whispered, "I told you I met someone else."

41

I think now is a good time to explain how my body is affected by my CP. My left side is more affected, but my right side has more intense spasticity. As Ken was making googly eyes at his new girlfriend, I lost my mind. My spastic right hand flew up and was hitting everything in sight. I think I said every four-letter word in the book, and then made up some new ones. Although it can sometimes be difficult to understand my speech with my CP accent, people tell me that when I curse, the words come out perfectly. The security men, there to protect the performers, had the unenviable job of carrying out of the gym a temporarily insane, squawking, flailing woman, while my faithful friend Denise, greatly embarrassed, drove my scooter behind them.

After that event, I paid Ken a visit. His roommate escorted me back to my dorm. I could not be mad at him because he knew what had been going on. He was in a tough spot, and he liked me better than The Other Woman. A couple of months later, I learned that The Other Woman was pregnant with Ken's child.

It took me five years to fully get over my first sexual love. It was a clunky step up my metaphorical staircase. Interestingly, this time the climb involved two disabled people; it wasn't the able-bodied world putting negative labels on me. I was a jilted woman. That stunk; although I now know it was for the best. In 1998, Ken was at Ramapo College, and I went to see him. He was recording in the very same studio. We went out to dinner that night and said good-bye in a civil manner. That night brought closure to our love affair and healing to my broken heart.

I bet you're wondering how the hell did I end up at Ramapo College anyway? The story isn't as juicy as the last one, but it *is* worth telling. As I sit here, looking at the multiple degrees on my living room wall, I'm laughing ironically to myself—in contrast to the intense anger that I still feel about the discouragement I encountered as I innocently began my journey into the wilds of higher education. Preview to coming attractions, below.

After obtaining my driver's license, driving around with my friends, kissing in the back seat with Fred, and living that dual life, I boldly decided that I wanted to go away to college for Business Administration/ Computer Science. I applied to two colleges, Rider and Ramapo, and was accepted at both. I distinctly remember the acceptance letter from Rider. It arrived on a Saturday morning. My parents were away, and I had had a big party the night before. I had gotten really drunk, and I think I kissed two guys. Trisha (from cooking class) was upstairs and yelled down, "You got a letter from Rider, and it's a big package." In those days, we did not have email, so a big package contained all the application materials and meant that you had been accepted to the school. I had been accepted to Rider University, the school of my dreams. You can just imagine how I felt.

A few days later, my mom and I went to visit. It was a breathtaking campus with a glistening pond. The first interview was with the Director of Student Affairs. That conversation was very positive, and she said she was looking forward to working with me to make some changes for accessibility and other issues. I was so excited; this was indeed *my* university. After that interview, I had another meeting with a Learning Specialist on campus. From the very first second I met her, I knew that this was not going to be one of the most positive experiences in my life. I told her that I had already been accepted to Rider, and my mom and I had some questions regarding accommodations. She inquired, "Are you *sure* you were accepted to Rider? You know this is a prestigious university. Maybe a two-year college would suit you better." *What?* That was the first time in my life that I had experienced educational discrimination directly due to my disability. I sobbed all the way home.

During that long drive, tears falling from my eyes, my crestfallen mom had no words to say, and we drove in silence. I declared, "She must be right, Mom. She has a PhD!"

Mom looked over at me and replied glumly, "Maybe she is right. Who knows?" Obviously Mom was as shocked as I was.

I continued to sob all night, but I didn't really know why I was so sad. Now when I or other people experience a shitty event in their lives, I can honestly see it as a growth experience. I don't believe in karma because that's too generous for the other person. Let me explain. Even though I grew positively from this and other ugly experiences in my life, I do not think the bad guys involved deserve good karma credit, too. You know, the bullshit that "Your tormentor is your teacher," and "It's all good." Yeah, right. By the same token, I don't wish ill or bad karma on anyone; that takes too much of *my* energy. Just get out of my life, and I'll carry on without you, thanks anyway.

I did carry on with my life, but *that* learning experience, I will always have with me. And it is one I share with all of my students: *Never equate education or degrees with intelligence.* My experience is that American culture is fixated on how many degrees a person has accumulated. As an overly zealous culture, we ignore everything else. I've seen how someone can have several degrees and still be one of the stupidest people around.

I decided I didn't want to go to Rider. Fuck 'em.

Shortly thereafter, I was accepted to Ramapo College with open arms.

Linden Hall. 108-B. That's where I resided for two years as an undergraduate at Ramapo College. It was my first-of-everything time. My first semester of college. First time getting high. First time having sex. First time realizing that people have sex all kinds of different ways, and at all times of the day. I remember going down the hallway of the dorm at noon and distinctly hearing groaning sexual noise behind someone's door. In my pre-college days, I thought that you only had sex after dinner! You know, like Mike and Carol Brady, who got all those kids to bed and *then* got their groove on. I thought you only had sex when two people were alone in the room. Oh, no! Roommates at college have sex with boyfriends or girlfriends lots of times of the day and/or night, in private or not.

This was also the first time I saw that I was prejudiced toward people with different sexual orientations. Or perhaps I just had a great deal of naiveté. I had a personal care attendant who helped me to dress, among other things. I found out that she was bisexual, which unnerved me. It also surprised and unnerved me to learn of my own prejudice! Ken told me to be professional about it. I was, and she was, and we're still good friends.

Before college, as a teenager, I did not know the extent and history of discrimination against African Americans. I finally saw it when I had honest conversations with my African American classmates outside Ramapo classrooms. I am hesitant to tell you about my former biases, due to my profession. You know I am a liberal professor of Disability

Studies working in an integrated academic setting. But back then I was prejudiced toward people of different sexual orientations as well as African Americans. I was woefully misguided and definitely wrong.

Back to my first semester at Ramapo College. I barely remember my classes, but I do remember my First Year Seminar class because the room was so noisy. We had to move our rambunctious class to Linden Lounge on the first floor. The second class I remember was Intro to Sociology with Dr. Lee. I recall this class because Ken walked me to the room just after we had had sex. It was wonderful sitting in class, dreaming about my infatuation. In addition to my daydreams, I remember being assigned a five-page research paper on a topic of our choice. I chose to do mine on *The Americans with Disabilities Act.*

The Office of Specialized Services played a major role in my freshman and sophomore years at Ramapo College. I really don't know why it's called "specialized services." In the discipline of Disability Studies, Dr. Litton states that the word "special" is condescending. What they're offering is not "specialized services," it's "disability services." The current name implies inequality, while "disability services" implies empowerment and equality. For example, UC Berkeley entitled their program "Disability Services"; they were the first in the nation to have such a program in the early 1960s.

In order to do the Sociology paper, my academic counselor from OSS, Barbara Wexler, hired a person to help me with my research. This man remains a very special soul in my life; I deeply loved and respected him.

You know when you go through your daily life, and you're in that mode of routine? You only think about your family and your close loved ones. So many people enter and exit your life; you simply can't remember everyone. However, if an individual enters and exits your life in a brilliant yet subtle way, he infiltrates your thoughts both consciously and unconsciously forevermore. Such a person can have a profound impact on your life. Such was the assistant for my ADA paper, despite the fact that I've forgotten his last name.

Ms. Wexler provided me with an incredible grandfather figure, an archetype both he and I were constantly aware of. He assisted me with the paper; however, I recall little of the details of the actual paper. What I vividly remember are our heartfelt conversations in his little red car, driving twenty miles per hour below the speed limit, and discussing family, love, and relationships. Doesn't it sound like a Hallmark moment, like *Tuesdays with Morrie?* Actually, my book was *Friday Afternoons with Ed.*

He loved his wife so much, and she was dying. He took me to see her a few times in Spring Valley, New York. Her name was Ruth, and they were so sweet together. I just hope that Mac and I have the same sweetness in our golden years.

On the way home, Ed and I usually talked about my life. It was so peculiar, exiting one scene of a play and entering another. And let me tell you, the scenes changed in ten seconds from PG à la *Tuesdays with Morrie* to X-rated sex, drugs, and rock 'n' roll!

I strolled into my dorm. "Hey man, what's up?" called the Resident Assistant, checking my college ID.

I'd always smile a sly, Friday-night smile and greet her with, "Nothing, Homey. Homey, don't play that." This was a rudely funny reference to a popular TV show at the dorm, *In Living Color.*

I went to my dorm room, the pungent aroma of pot emanating from all the other rooms. I reached Denise Connor's room. (To this day, she remains an enduring pal, with whom I speak about three times weekly.) With impunity, I swung open the door and demanded, "What's the story for tonight?"

Now I must explain, I have never, ever seen Denise smoke or get drunk or high. I'm amazed that we've remained friends all these years.

"You know I don't do the stuff you do!"

"Okay, I'll tell you what. You do your thing, and lemme do mine."

"Yeah, sure. All those things that people with disabilities *don't* do!"

"Who, me?"

"No, your able-bodied twin!"

So I went to the apartments on campus to drink and, because I was underage, tried to stay out of trouble. That's where all the upperclassmen lived, and it was riotous. After getting my groove on and imbibing rum and coke with a straw, I returned to my dorm, somewhat tipsy, and asked, "What time is Stateline open till?"

It wasn't apparent that I was tipsy, so my roommate and I decided to go to the Stateline Diner, even though it was about 3:30 in the morning. For the potato skins with the extra sour cream. This constituted a typical Friday night that first semester on campus. Basically, it was sheer adolescent heaven.

What? How did I fare academically? The poor disabled girl, who was strongly advised to consider options other than a four-year college? I always did very well and graduated with a 3.7 GPA, which made me an "A" student. Not bad. I was not unlike many other students, with or without disabilities. My early college years actually contributed more to my social and emotional growth than to my academic growth. Contrary to that Rider specialist's advice, I eventually fit right into collegiate life. I knew that I'd fit in, and I certainly know it now as a successful professor.

I'm sure you've been given bad advice at some time in your life, so I bet you can relate. In that way (and in many others), you and I are way more alike than we are different. Thus, from that universal point of view, we all have our staircases of oppression. For me, the staircase is omnipresent, sometimes obviously so, sometimes not. I have several defenses against that damn staircase. The most effective are my major accomplishments, my sense of humor, and my compassion—especially with my students. Keep reading–you can be the judge of my interpersonal compassion.

From time to time you've read how I refer to "my staircase of oppression." This is meant to serve as a reminder, to me and to my readers, of its omnipresence. Fortunately, I'm competitive, tenacious, and determined. Because of this, I am able to keep climbing that staircase. Whether by nature or nurture or both, that's who I am—and that's always been a good thing.

Saturdays, I usually hung low and did some studying. Sundays, I went home, only to realize that my childhood really hadn't been as great as it had once seemed. My young adult consciousness was beginning to blossom, and I was starting to rebel against my conservative upper-middle class background. My parents were wondering what the hell was going on. For that matter, *I* was wondering what the hell was going on. Something did not quite fit, and it became apparent to me on my Sunday visits.

To illustrate our changing relationship, here's an analogy. Mac always hates when I open a bottle of Diet Coke and a bottle of water simultaneously. Invariably, I leave the caps off both bottles, and neat freak that he is, he can't stand it. In the dark kitchen after he comes home from work, while I'm snoozing soundly, he attempts to make the caps fit. In his weary stupor, he always confuses the wrong bottle with the wrong cap. Sometimes they fit, but not quite right, and not really. This nightly occurrence reminds me of my relationship with my family during my freshman year at Ramapo . . . and, in truth, for a number of years to come.

Presently, in addition to teaching Disability Studies, I teach First Year Seminar. As I see the leaves turn color each autumn, I see my freshmen students becoming adults. I witness my students rebelling against their parents, and I endeavor to help them transition into young adulthood. Although I make an honest effort to do this, I truly feel that my role as "mentor for transition into adulthood" is bullshit–because no one can "ease" anyone into self-exploration and self-understanding. Nonetheless, you gotta do what you gotta do to make money. Perhaps I'm being cynical or self-deprecating about my role as teacher and mentor because I've had several terrific mentors in my life, and my students recently nominated me for Professor of the Year at Ramapo. That's meaningful to me. Despite this, I believe that the bulk of self-exploration emanates from within. Its very nature is innate.

In my First Year Seminar class, my requirements are for students to probe life memories in a chronological fashion by writing a series of papers to capture them. The papers are eight in number and follow Erikson's Life Development Stages. I ask the students to take a scholarly approach to self-exploration, as well as to exploring their relationships with others.

(Speaking of relationships, as I'm writing my poor husband is having a hard time putting on the bottle caps I carelessly left off last night. He grumbles and calls me "Lucy," but we still have a good relationship. He will always be my sweet "Ricky.")

Anyway, back to my rebellious weekends at home. Truthfully, I don't remember much of the minutiae of those weekends. All I know is that being back home presented a very different and restrictive lifestyle from the dorms. Can you imagine coming from a pot-infested hallway, young people moaning and groaning in heated sexual ecstasy behind dorm doors—only to arrive in the now-foreign planet of my childhood home, where you could a hear a pin drop? I saw no possible intersection of my two worlds.

Like Eddie Murphy in *Coming to America*, I was treated as beloved royalty in my parents' traditional domain, which was an upper-middle class, oh-so-right-wing existence. At college, I was a young rebel, ready to face the world with my newfound bold left-wing views. I realize that right wing/left wing is unrealistic bullshit because each issue in politics is separate. Sweeping generalizations about social policy and ideology are far too simplistic. Remember, once upon a time both the abolition of slavery and a woman's right to vote were considered radical left-wing ideas. I can easily expound on this right wing/left wing bullshit, but I prefer that you, the reader, take as long as you like pondering this existential, sociopolitical quandary.

Eventually I achieved a mutually respectful relationship with my parents. No matter what shit was going on (and there has been a lot!), our love has always tethered us.

However, every once in a while my childhood life and my college life came to a lightning bolt intersection. The week after Thanksgiving 1993, I learned that my first sexual love, Ken, had broken my heart. In reaction, I was looking for a physical bond with someone. So I called a guy from high school, named Dave, for whom I had always had the hots. He decided to come to Ramapo and get drunk with me in my dorm room. We put a case of beer in my little refrigerator. (Well, not exactly. The fridge was owned by Ramapo, and was so damn small we could only stick six beers in it at a time. So when you opened the fridge, all you could see were cans of Bud Light.) Dan and I decided to go to the upperclassmen apartments to kick off our drunken buzz. Unfortunately, Dave met another woman and hooked up with her—back in my dorm room, no less! Meanwhile, I was at the apartments fighting with Ken.

Back then we didn't have cell phones, and Denise was running frantically to the apartments, looking for me, drunk as I was.

"Chris, Security is in your room, along with the Assistant Dean of Students! Dave is in there with some white chick, making a lot of noise.

Security took all your beer, and the Assistant Dean of Students wants to see you tomorrow—Sunday morning at nine o'clock!"

"Whatever," I replied in my drunken stupor.

"'Whatever'? Are you crazy, woman? You're really drunk!"

The next morning, I was not intoxicated at all, but I was terrified. I recall that same morning I discovered a condom wrapper in the toilet. Thanks a lot, Dave. Anyway, I dressed and went to see the Assistant Dean of Students, who, believe it or not, is my mentor today, and recently, I was his Teaching Assistant...but that all happened years later, and on that fateful Sunday in November, 1993, it felt like my DOOMSDAY!

I'd like to digress to my current professional relationship with the esteemed Dr. Patrick Chang, former Assistant Dean of Students, today Vice Provost of Academic Technology. With mutual respect, we sit together at professional meetings. Everyone's demeanor at these important meetings, including Dr. Chang's and mine, is sober, committed, and dedicated. Quite often, as we exit after adjournment, Dr. Chang and I joke casually and affectionately.

"Hi, Dr. McCohnell."

(Dr. Chang is always encouraging me to go back for my doctoral degree, and that is his subtle way of reminding me—of course, using my new married name. More about the glorious wedding later.)

I usually refer to Dr. Chang as precisely that, "Dr. Chang," to recognize his accomplishments at the college. After these intros, he jokes and says:

"I still have one of your old beers."

"Those beers are ancient. If I drink one now, I'd probably keel over."

Back at Doomsday, I never would have thought *that* conversation could have happened. After all, I was nineteen years old and in deep, dreadful shit.

"Come in, Miss Komoroski."

Dr. Chang was behind the desk, wearing a black suit and tie. I entered the room on my scooter very nervously and hit another chair in the room by accident.

I blurted instantly, "I'm sorry, Dr. Chang!" And I was.

What my deluded mind heard in response was, "I could call your Mommy and Daddy! And I could kick you off campus!"

You wanna know what really happened? Okay, I'm sure he said something somewhat similar in an extremely professional manner; nevertheless, the consequences for my outrageous behavior left me elated and willing to do whatever he demanded.

I scooted out of his office, rejoicing to myself, "I am *not* kicked off campus, and *all* I need to do is Community Service! And Mommy and Daddy are not going to find out!"

After that cataclysmic meeting, I went to see my faithful friend, Denise. I told her my good news. Soon afterward, in a bout of guilt, I returned somberly to my dorm room to call Stevie.

I really felt awful about the whole incident, and I needed to tell some member of my family. Stevie and I were the closest at the time, so I chose him. I called him up, nervous, as any younger sibling would be. I recounted the whole story, and know what he did? He laughed at me and said, "That's it? Ha! Don't worry"

The next thing I knew, my mother and my beloved grandfather called me, and Grandpa was angry with me because I had wasted a case of perfectly good beer, which he could have used for his weekly poker games with his buddies. I honestly do not remember what Mommy said or inferred. I guess that she and the whole family were glad that I was right on target in my emotional and behavioral maturation. So was I.

During that winter break, Trisha and I were together a lot, trying to assuage my hurt feelings about Ken. I was pissed off that Ken had abandoned me for an ugly–in my opinion--woman. When I returned to campus in late January, I realized that I was even more pissed at Ken than I had originally thought, so I deliberately started to date a geek out of spite. Just imagine, last year I had been sleeping with the coolest guy on campus, and now I was dating the biggest geek on campus.

While Ken was preparing to be a father in NYC, I was getting the third degree from all my nosy friends.

"Tipsy K, why in the heck are you dating that geek?"

"Because I'm in love!"

"Too bad your true love is in NYC, and he's with someone else."

"Yeah, yeah, shut up, asshole."

All of my freshman buddies on campus hated Ken. Me, too...well, kinda. But I had no one else, or so I thought.

Next, I decided to join a fraority, which is a co-ed sorority. The pledging was the longest two months of my life. They told me exactly what to wear, how to wear it, what to do, the usual hazing bullshit. However, I could find something great in every yucky scenario of the hazing. In my first pledge class, there were five of us: four young women and one young man. And guess who I quickly befriended? The young man. His name was Rick. He was the most laid-back human being I had ever met in my youth. We both abhorred pledging. The other people in our pledge class were gung ho. I really wanted to get my supposedly important Phi Kappa Delta letters, so I was begrudgingly playing along. Rick, on the other hand, didn't do a thing to receive his letters, so I had to frequently kick him in his royal ass.

A chilly weekend in November turned out to be our Hell Week. We were gonna cross over to PKD membership, but we were gonna have to experience torture first. Rick forgot his mandatory paddle. If you don't know what that implies, ask someone in a Greek fraternity or fraority, or watch *Animal House*. Our pledge leader decided to drive in a torrential downpour to get a freakin' paddle for Rick. Guess who drove all of us? As many friends and relatives have declared over the years, "Only you, Christine." Well, my driving scared the shit out of all of them because I was so pissed at Rick that I ran over a tall curb on purpose—full force!

Rick blurted, "What the hell are you doing, Sorry?" That was one of my other nicknames.

"Getting your freakin' paddle, Slacker!"

"Please, be quiet, and please, please, get us there safe," bleated one of the terrified young women in the back seat. They were all at my mercy.

"Whenever Slacker and Sorry are in the same room, or in this case, the same car, it's chaos! God help us," chimed in another petrified passenger.

Believe it or not, we crossed over safely within twenty-four hours and became proud PKD members. After finally crossing over, however, I realized that these people were not my real friends after all. This was bullshit. During Hell Week, they were all playing baseball in hurricane-strong rain and decided to have me sit there in the downpour and simply watch the shenanigans. If that wasn't disability discrimination, I don't know what was. In fact, often during those early college years, when I wanted to be fully accepted in a social situation, I got turned down or marginalized. Each time, I felt like shit. After all, I had brains, a sense of humor, a sense of adventure, *and* I was trying to climb the rickety old staircase of oppression.

At that period of my life, I was not too fond of words that started with the letter "g." You know, like Greek or geek . . . or God. Eventually, I would find and embrace Buddhism, but as a young college student, spirituality was the last thing on my mind. My relationship with the Almighty was vastly unclear to me in my early twenties, and the strict dogma of religion was out of the question. That was how it remained for a long time. To be continued.

One night as I rolled into my teeny room, I saw the light blinking on my answering machine, and my sense of adventure returned. I was still physically infatuated with Ken. I hoped excitedly that maybe he had left a message for me. Back in those days, answering machines were pretty new. You had to totally rewind the tape to listen to messages. I was waiting anxiously as the machine rewound, and I was getting excited. But my lust cooled down immediately when I heard the message. It was my counselor from Specialized Services requesting that I call her back. I said, to myself, "Dammit. Did they find me drinking again?" Of course I had been drinking again. In fact I was tipsy as I was listening to the damn message!

I called her back the next day. She suggested that I apply to an institute in Minnesota, which had a focus on empowering college students with disabilities. Trusty Ms. Wexler, who had paired me with my beloved ADA grandfather, actually saw potential in me. I had been oblivious to my own potential and empowerment. I was twenty years old. At this unexpected moment, I began to glimpse azure sky far above the staircase.

I've come to see that as we go through life, we often do not realize what we're doing until we write it down. As I've said, while writing my memoirs, I've discovered that every five years something major has occurred in my life. The momentous milestone of my trip to Minnesota at age twenty truly helped me to identify myself as an empowered woman with a disability.

Together, Ms. Wexler and I applied to the institute and were accepted. We took a flight on August 1, 1994, and during the flight, I realized that I was becoming an adult. In one week's time, I couldn't fully grasp the transformation that was happening to me. I must say that it was certainly one of the most powerful weeks in my life. A whole new world was unfolding right before my eyes. I was experiencing Disability History and Disability Pride. Blossoming empowerment was growing within. Yes, all this was in my subconscious, trickling into my consciousness during my time in Minnesota and beyond, but, in true fashion, I was also busy trying to hang out with a cute guy I met. We students worked diligently during the day, but at night about twenty of us in wheelchairs went to a bar. The bartender was used to us by the last night. The conference was one of the high points of my life, and on August 6, 1994, I announced to the entire group of twenty-eight people that I was a *proud* woman with a disability.

I still see Ms.Wexler on the Ramapo campus, and I often forget that she was the one who helped me to identify myself. I guess what I'm trying to say is a public *thank you* to Ms. Wexler.

"Oh, shit." My cell phone is ringing as I'm speeding on my way to Ramapo, and I have to pull over. I know it's Mac because I have a special ring for him. I should have never stopped for that damn Starbucks. Shit.

"I found a really good deal," he chirps cheerfully.

"Honey, just buy the damn thing, whatever it is! I'm late already!"

"Well, if you would leave on time and not stop for Starbucks, you wouldn't be late." (Now how does he know I stopped for Starbucks? He knows everything. Dammit.)

Too bad I didn't meet Mac at Starbucks in Minnesota in 1994. While I was at the institute, he was working at the hospital right down the street. Oftentimes, when we are lying in bed, I ask him, "Why didn't we meet *before* your first marriage? Like in Minnesota, in 1994?"

His astute reply is, "We weren't ready for this relationship." He's right because back then I yearned to sow my wild oats. And I did.

At this point, I'd like to go into more detail about my profound experiences at the institute. It provided me with a different perspective on disability and the ideology that the able-bodied world had forced on me. Because of Medical Model values, I had never been exposed to the rich history and culture of people with disabilities. Why had my previous educators been teaching me everything *except* the momentous legislation concerning people with disabilities, which would have surely motivated me to become a disability rights teacher and activist? To me, it makes great sense to teach young people with disabilities that they have a proud culture and heritage. In fact, that's why I am somewhat indifferent about inclusion education, mainly because of *the utter lack of knowledge of disability history* that the vast majority of teachers have. Inclusion is not the problem, but the prejudicial notion that "we don't want anyone to feel they have a disability" discounts the *importance* of Disability Pride. We do not want to be our able-bodied peers, or even appear to be. Include us—in everything–but please don't make our disabilities pejorative. I must repeat myself: People with disabilities have a rich, proud history and culture.

I'm sure that everyone knows that Thomas Edison invented the first practical light bulb, but I bet your teachers never told you (they never told me) that he had a disability. Did you know that Galileo had a disability, and so did Beethoven, Nelson Rockefeller, and Bud Abbott (of Abbott and Costello fame)? How about Milton, Goya, Churchill, Newton, Einstein? Woodrow Wilson, Ed Sullivan, Whoopi Goldberg, and Bruce Jenner? Do you know who Harriet Tubman was? I bet you have no idea why I connect with Harriet Tubman on a heartfelt level. She had a pronounced disability (narcolepsy) due to multiple beatings from her slave owner. I connect with her on a disability level, as well as connecting on an anti-slavery level.

When I married Mac on the afternoon of June 4, 2006, we decided to "jump over the broom"—just as slaves had done when they "married" before the Civil War. It was strictly prohibited by law for African American slaves to wed. Remember, my beloved husband is African American, with a slave heritage. It was a true symbol of our love and history, and can you imagine me with my spastic CP jumping over a freakin' broom?! Well, it was quite a sight. It was a fantastic wedding. We love and respect each other very much, and it was most evident during our vows and jubilant celebration afterward—when, naturally, we danced the night away. Mac and I also slow danced to "The Love of my Life," and we put *Dancing with the Stars* to shame when the up tempos roused the happy crowd to boogie-oogie-woogie on down with us. My ninety-two-year-old mother-in-law even joined in the dancing jubilation. The whole happy roomful engaged in frenzied, nonstop feasting as they boogied the night away with Mac and me at the groovy helm. With or without my walker, I am a hot, joyous dancer, if I say so myself. In fact, everyone said as much. It was fantastic! Both my mom and dad had walked me down the aisle, each supporting me by my arms. I didn't use a walker until they gave me away at the blossom-festooned altar. My friends tell me there was not a dry eye in the gorgeous, flower-laden banquet room at the Summit Hotel, where we were pronounced husband and wife. It was perfect.

However, at the age of twenty, my sophomore year in college, I thought that I would never, ever get married. Never! I innocently believed that I would marry the first man I had sex with, but that was not to be because as I've already said, Ken got another girl pregnant, and they didn't even wed. Reality came in full force then. It was not until seven years later that I met a man I considered marrying. I bet you're just dying to know who he was (it wasn't yet Mac), but you'll just have to keep reading to find out. Ha ha! I love a good story with unexpected zigs and zags. Trust me, those sharp turns have been the saga of my life—for better or worse.

Back then in 1994 and 1995, my peers and my academic work at Ramapo were definitely not on my priority list. During that school year, my siblings all had major problems. I'd like to go into some detail about my relationships with them, so here are my youthful perceptions of each sibling, as well as of my mother figure.

Until the age of about six, I had always thought that I had two mothers. The reason for my belief was due to the difficulties and the amount of the care I needed. That burden fell primarily on Mom and Kim, and thus my mother's and my sister's love merged into a maternal love for me. My first memory of my sister Kim was not at all based on her lovely physical presence, but on her wild hot pink '70s wallpaper! She had a big canopy bed, and boy-oh-by was it difficult for me to climb aboard. When at last I had clambered onto her pretty bed, I pretended to be a breathtaking (and now breathless) princess, waving elegantly to my abundant, adoring fans right under Kim's lacy canopy. Sometimes I was an ace spy. Sometimes I was just hangin' out with my beloved Elmo in a special spot reserved just for us.

But I have to confess that most of the above paragraph is a wistful fabrication. With my spastic CP, I was never able to climb onto her bed. I only dreamed of those scenarios. Family and friends had to hoist me up on that fanciful bed—not nearly as fun as my wishful thinking, but not too bad.

One day, after Kim had set me on her bed, she tiptoed excitedly into the bathroom, announcing that she was going to fix my make-up like a big girl. Wow!! But, as usual, I had a secret agenda. While she was in the bathroom gathering various toiletries, I peeked under her bed and was delighted to find a Play Doh Factory! I just knew that Kim was getting that gift for me for Christmas. I was overjoyed and couldn't believe my eyes, but smart Kim discovered my sneaky ways.

You know how she found out? I told her myself, but that was because she caught me as a Peeping Tom . . . so I had to confess, naturally.

"That Play Doh Station is for your friend Kelly."

That was the very first time that I actually got caught doing something naughty, which resulted in my feeling yucky. Yet, I must admit, if Kim were here with me today and read this particular part of the story, she would just shrug. She'd tell you my mischief had begun long before that event and continued long after. I was a handful.

My sister would spend much time with me acting as my "second" mommy. I sometimes consider the generosity and unconditional love my sister bestowed upon me as odd. If I had been her, I would have been intensely jealous of the fact that much of the love in the household was now shifting to this new human being—baby me—just about seven years Kim's junior. Despite any jealousy, she took good care of me, and I treasured every single moment of time with my Mommy Number Two.

What do I say about Steven? To describe our relationship is simple. I cried my eyes out to my mommy because Stevie had a girlfriend—and it wasn't me!

"Honey, you can't marry your brother," my mom said soothingly.

"Waa! Why not? Waa!"

Stevie would take me everywhere. We were best buddies.

My parents used to take Stevie and me to Club Med, and there, we danced every night away at the disco. The young women would always give me strange looks until they found out that I was his sister. After that, they immediately became my best friends. I wonder why? As a little kid, I admired Stevie just as the women at Club Med did. He was my knight in shining armor.

As for my brother Charlie, who was the oldest of us four, we never got along. He knew just how to push my buttons ever since I emerged from the womb. Charlie is one of my mom's favorites to this day. I don't really remember him much when I was growing up. I do remember that his former bedroom had been converted into my accessible bedroom and bathroom because it was so large. My mom was no longer able to pick me up and bathe me, but I could now do it myself because the bathroom was accessible. (Am I repeating myself here? After all, I am "Lucy.") We were fortunate to have the means to have the accessible bathroom built, but a large room was needed, so Charlie unwillingly surrendered his bedroom.

Back when it had been his room, it was very dark, adjacent to my parents' bedroom. I clearly recall crawling very fast to my nursery because I thought there was a ghost in there. In addition, Charlie had live snakes in his room. (That's why I had the oldest living goldfish around. Remember what I said before about my goldfish? I think that's creepy, too.)

Charlie has rarely exhibited emotion, but he is the most internally emotional person in the whole family. He portrays himself as a bully, but my brother is a sensitive guy. Okay, my husband has him beat in the sensitivity department, but either way, both men are buttercups.

Charlie is a most intelligent guy. He knows just about every fact in the whole wide world; you can ask him anything, and he'll respond knowledgeably. However, he does not conform to or comply with authority. Actually, there is so much to share about Charlie, but it's not fair for me to speak about it.

It is my belief that his true love was his first wife Traci. She became a part of my life when I was eleven years old. We are both absolutely casual about fashion and appearance and definitely lean toward adventures of all types.

Traci and I had nicknames for each other; she called me, "Mickey" and I called her "Fickey." One time, we were hanging out at her old house in Linden, New Jersey, with an odd friend of hers. And he was odd, let me tell you. He was stoned all the time, so I never knew what he was going to do or say. He informed us that when you watch R-rated movies on TV, instead of using the word "motherfucker," the censors use the words "Mickey" and "Fickey." Thus, the birth of our nicknames!

Over time, Traci and I developed a close bond. In fact, at my wedding, she came up to me and said, "I'm so proud of you, Mickey."

"Thank you, Fickey."

Some of my wildest times, like getting kicked out of rowdy bars, were with my beloved Fickey.

Charlie and Traci made three beautiful kids. The middle child, Jamie Lee, is my godchild and was my junior bridesmaid. Every time she looks at me with her big brown eyes, my heart just melts. Mac and I have decided not to have any children and Jamie is the closest soul who represents a daughter to me. CJ is the youngest of the three and the only blood-related nephew. He is cute as a button. Kelsi, the oldest, reminds me of my youthful babysitter, and I relate to her the best due to the profound connectedness I have with adolescents.

At the same time, a part of me cannot attach to young children. I guess that's because of the anger I have because I cannot produce a child, and so my soul lacks true empathy with small children. Numerous people think that Mac and I would produce beautiful children, but I seriously doubt that will come true. So instead we take many wonderful vacations to make up for the fact that there are no children of our own in our lives. In fact, Mac has a son, Jason, who is twenty-six years old and Jason has a three-year-old daughter. The baby's name is Nevaeh, which is "heaven" spelled backwards. Just think, I am a stepmom to a grown man and a step-grandma to a preschooler, and I'm only in my early thirties!

When I was a little younger than Jason, at the tender age of twenty, which hits that fateful five-year marker, our family was enduring crisis after crisis. It seemed as if the bad luck was never going to end. Stevie and the rest of the family experienced a major loss in our lives. I have never forgotten the chilly day in October, 1994, a Sunday to be exact, when a friend of the family came crying hysterically to my mom, sobbing that her older brother had killed himself. He had gone to a wedding with his wife, and they had an argument. He came back to his mother's house, the house right next door to ours, and decided to play Russian roulette. He lost. I guess that friend really thought of my mom as her mom because I distinctly remember my mom holding her for three hours just like a mother hugging her baby. My brother Stevie was screaming downstairs in the basement where she and I had played house together. And you know what? I can't even remember where I was in the house because that raw emotion had a hideous and surreal effect on everyone. At the funeral, I held my brother's hand through the whole ordeal. I never saw him cry so much in my life. His friend's suicide took a great toll on him.

Nowadays, I talk to many different people during my daily routine, which includes a certain amount of bullshit. I hear a lot of "Money can solve everything." I really don't understand how people believe that stupid notion. Maybe they believe it because they want to achieve some ultimate "Midas" goal, and they think money can purchase it for them. Money could not fix the pain and grief that Stevie's friend and his shattered family endured. I don't think that money will ever lift that horrendous pain and sorrow.

Later in 1995, I began my career path. Back then I just thought that I was training to be a Peer Facilitator, a big-deal job on campus. Ramapo College requires that students take a course in their first year to acclimate themselves to the college setting. Currently, I teach First Year Seminar, but I had to start somewhere. For me, that was in the educational arena as a Peer Facilitator (a teacher's assistant who helps the busy professor). To lay a solid foundation as a promising facilitator, you have to take a class on the dynamics of the job. During that spring semester, I took the course.

Remember Rick and the freakin' paddle? Well, Rick and I got "accepted" into the course. I remember the classroom—one that no longer exists. There were fifteen of us. The first part of the semester, we learned about Ramapo. The second part, we learned about each other. We all thought we were freakin' royalty, and we were! Rick and I became inseparable. But the funny thing was we never had sex or even so much as made out. I was dating a man who was living off campus, a real character. It just so happened that he was a member of an African

American fraternity on campus. I had met him at a dance in the student center where the dancing was much dirtier than in *Dirty Dancing*. I was engaging in this wild dancing with my partner, who was a great dancer and also gay. Rashad, who was soon to be my off-campus man, saw me and started to talk to me.

"Hey, you dance pretty damn good. But my best friend is dating your gay partner."

"Yeah, I know," I retorted. "Better not blow my f'in cover!"

One thing led to another, and Rashad and I became more than friends. Maybe less than friends, but more physical. Yeah, now that I think about it, Rashad and I had a deep connection, and it was purely affectionate. Rashad was on campus due to his role in his fraternity. He was the Pledge Master, and boy, was he in charge. Reminiscing about Rashad, I have to say he should win an Oscar. He could imitate me so perfectly that I wondered if our affection had actually transferred some CP DNA into his body. It was really, really hilarious. He could imitate my up-pointed CP toe to a T, as well as my CP accent and my wise-ass attitude. Look out, Jamie Foxx!

During Pledge Week, Rashad had two pledges sit in front of him as he was riotously imitating me. They were not allowed to laugh or make a sound. I got to watch, and it was so funny! If they laughed or made a sound of any kind, their punishment was that they had to run across campus clothed only in their underwear in the freezing cold to get me a straw for my tequila! I still laugh when I remember it because they each guffawed despite their struggle not to. So they each had to disrobe and run. Or I should say, one guy ran, the other guy rolled in his wheelchair—in his underwear. When the two of them reached the other side of the campus, they had a helluva time finding a straw. When they finally "crossed over," they were furious and said that they would have rather been beaten than been outside in their underwear that frigid February.

My brief affair with Rashad had an indelible impact on my life. To this day, I find the hardest thing to do is to hold in a big belly laugh. I challenge you to try—there's nothing like it, and you will not succeed.

During the spring semester that year, I was active in my Peer Facilitator class, and was hanging out with Rick. I became friends with the woman down the hall. Her name was also Tracey, and we talked about everything. She was very conservative, like Denise, and I was the wild one who came home drunk, while Tracey and Denise giggled and made fun of me.

That summer, my family and I vacationed in North Carolina. We went away with the Stavitski clan. As you recall, the Stavitskis have always been like family to us. Everything was fine, calm, and status quo. During that summer, I had a dated a guy who was exactly like Charlie. He got on my nerves all the time, and he smelled horrendously too!

Speaking of encounters, I almost forgot to mention that during the winter break my PCA and I went on a Club Med vacation, one of the most raucous of my life. We were in the heavenly Turks and Caicos Islands, and we got completely plastered every night of our vacation— eight nights straight. I am damn lucky that in a few years, I was able to simply stop that kind of partying and drinking, I know people who struggle to stop. It was easy for me. Go figure. But, as I have said, I developed my own rotten issues later on.

One night, I woke up with a guy right next to me in bed. I highly doubt that I had sex with him—we were both fully dressed! But then again, I wouldn't bet my life on it. I remember that one of my friends, Judy, who was also on this vacation and is bisexual, was trying oh so diligently to get some woman to have sex with her.

We were all wild young people. In addition to my questionable one-night stand, I met a guy on the beach. My advice to people who are unable to walk, especially young women, is *never* go on a beach with a man you barely know. In my case, this man forced himself on me, but I was fortunate because I was able to stop him from doing anything. He backed off, and I got off the beach!

That vacation was one of the best weeks of my life because of the outrageously wild, carefree fun we experienced. My idea of fun today is relaxing at home with Mac. I just love occasionally watching a movie as we sit on our luscious two-person La-Z-Boy recliner. Buddhism and Zen. Boy, have times changed for the better.

As I go speeding down 202 with my Starbucks coffee in its holder, I'm thinking to myself, *Why can't we just buy a house closer to Ramapo?* This damn commute is getting longer and longer to me. Then I remember that my husband works at Princeton Hospital. If you don't know New Jersey, that means that we dwell equidistant from our jobs; plus, Mommy and Daddy are only twenty minutes away. My mind wanders back to the fact that Mac's cell call had somewhat uninvitingly interrupted my trip down Memory Lane with you. I wonder what's such a big deal that he had to call. I guess I'll find out tonight.

I'm now ten minutes late, and I'm in the Ramapo parking lot. I cannot use an ID-coded card as eligibility for an accessible spot because my fine motor skills cannot and will not cooperate to let me swipe a key card. I am fortunate that almost all of the security guards know who I am, and they simply push a little button, and automatically the gate opens. No matter how late I am, I always wave and smile and say, "Don't work too hard!"

As I drive up to the parking lot, I get very discouraged about who is parking in the accessible spots. This is a valid concern regarding who is permitted to park in the lot for persons with disabilities, and who is not. It doesn't seem just when I see a student or any number of administrative personnel get out of a car in an accessible parking spot and run into the building. I need extra space to lower the van's ramp. If I don't have that extra space, I'm screwed. I'm late for a meeting, and there are no spots available. Sure enough, when I look around, I observe faculty, staff, and students getting out of their cars in the accessible parking area and running to the door because it's freezing cold outside. These people are not disabled, and they have parked illegally. Dammit to hell, I just don't understand that. Plus, I'm screwed.

One of the most provocative questions I ask my students is, "Are we ever really free of prejudging others?" The politically correct answer is, "Yes, of course." But as you can tell, this memoir is not exactly politically correct. My answer to that question is, "We are never free from prejudging others." In the parking lot, I am prejudging the Ramapo community. In fact, I have numerous prejudices that I keep to myself or share with Mac. You know why? Simply because I'm human. I am lucky because Mac is a safe haven for my feelings.

Speaking of feelings, I had mixed emotions about the first apartment I got on campus after I left the dorms. It was what you call a shotgun apartment, and a real shitty looking one at that. For example, I had to use a manual key to open the front door. Aaah, fine motor skills again. I had a big polka-dot ribbon tied around the knob so I could pull the door closed when I left. The apartment had indoor/outdoor carpeting, which had probably been there well over twenty years. To my right was a teeny little living room with wood furniture that had old pillows on it. Then there was an ugly coffee table with multiple stains on it, stemming from those twenty years of use. And yet, the whole apartment was the most wonderful place in the world to me because I could sleep on the couch and use the coffee table and spill stuff on the floor or furniture and not worry about staining anything. And it was all mine. Pure heaven.

Attached to the living area of my apartment was the kitchen area. One big conjoined room. No, make that one small conjoined room. Separating these rooms was a 3x3 foot area of linoleum, which indicated the "kitchen." I purchased a cheap stand from K-Mart to put my microwave on. In the middle of the linoleum was a wooden table for four people. I usually sat by the sink when I had friends over. An ugly 1969 refrigerator stood in the right corner. Next to that was the sink, with cabinets above and below. Of course there were also a 1969 stove and a 1969 oven. Sunday evenings, my mom would pack me up with groceries and wave good-bye for what she thought was going to be a week, but it was actually a month before I would see her again. The groceries were one helluva nuisance because I had a tiny fridge and neither counter space nor drying rack for my dishes. Why in the world would I want to leave my terrific apartment to go home every weekend?

When I did visit home, my drive back to school constituted speeding along the Garden State Parkway. Back then there was no E-Z Pass, just tokens you tossed into a basket as you went through the toll. "Oh, well, I missed the freakin' basket again," I would mutter. You'd think that I would just drive up to the tollbooth and hand over the damn token to the toll collector, but oh no, I was too cool for that. I just kept throwing the stupid tokens and missing the bucket. Later, as I pulled up to my apartment, I dreaded taking the groceries inside because the items, including my tampons, would constantly fall out of the bag! And then without fail a hot guy would walk by, pick them up, and say, "Here you go, Chris."

When I at last reached my lovely apartment, I would roll up the blinds to serve as entertainment for my neighbors, because I would invariably have to chip away at my icebox. The fridge was so small that the freezer was actually inside it, and with all the times the refrigerator was opened, more and more ice became encrusted in the icebox. So I would chip away at all the damn ice with a cheap knife, cursing at the top of my lungs. It was a comical sight, and that's how my neighbors knew I was home. But it gets funnier! My neighbors would come by and ask, "Do you need help, Tipsy K?"

"No, but I got beer, so come in and keep me company."

After I chipped away all the ice, I put my food in the freezer. Now think about it. What would be my next problem? As I chipped away the ice, the floor became soaking wet. So I walked around in wet socks, and that essentially was my lovely, peaceful Sunday afternoon.

Back to the description of my apartment. Straight through the dining/kitchen area was a bathroom. It had two doors, one that closed it off from the living/kitchen area and another that separated it from the bedroom. So you had to walk through the living/kitchen area *and* the bathroom to get to the bedroom. This limited privacy for anyone in any of those rooms!

On the right side of this fabulous bathroom was a sink, and on the left side were the toilet and the shower, with my shower chair protruding from it because the stall was so small. When you entered the bedroom, there were twin beds on either wall. (No, I did not have a roommate, hallelujah!) My bed was on the right side of the room, and it was the most comfortable bed I have ever slept on; however, each morning I would get virtually electrocuted by the metal box springs. This happened all year round, no matter what the season. I swear the joint was haunted!

Next to my bed was a cute end table that I bought at the same old K-Mart. (Back then they did not have Wal-Mart or IKEA in New Jersey.) Next to the end table, I had my computer; it was really just a word processor because there was no Internet and no email in those days. For you in the new generation, our entertainment consisted of watching MTV in the living room and talking on the phone with a freakin' cord attached. If you don't know what I'm describing, I'm sure your aged parents will be glad to tell you more about it. Also, I had only one phone jack in the apartment, and it was, of all places, in the bathroom! If you were in the bathroom and the phone rang, you answered with sound effects in the background. Get the picture?

There were lots of wild parties, and remember, I had two beds in that bedroom. And no one ever sat on *my* bed, or I would kick their ass. I was a typical college kid, I guess.

I hope you laughed as I described my apartment. To many people it would qualify as a dive, but to me, it was a true utopia.

In a few other ways, I was not a typical college student. As I have told you before, many people have encouraged me over the years to write my memoirs, so that I could at least try to educate people about the uninhibited life I've led, especially because I have a physical disability. Most people don't think that a young female with pronounced CP could possibly have a fun, wild, and crazy social life, and still be smart and motivated. In fact one of the most difficult relationships I've ever had involved one of my female personal care assistants, specifically because her expectations and perceptions of what I would be like were mistaken.

Initially, when people learn that I have a personal care assistant, they automatically think it is a glorious thing. Why not? A PCA does the laundry, helps clean the house, helps me get dressed, and makes my life a whole lot easier. In reality, having a PCA is the most difficult relationship anyone can have due to the level of intimacy that the PCA and the person with a disability share. Can you imagine having someone dress you and assist you with intimate needs, and then you find out that they're taking advantage of you by stealing from you or by cutting their hours in half and expecting full pay?

My junior year was not the happiest of my life because the PCA was horrible. I have many conversations with disabled peers about our PCAs, and unfortunately 99% of them have endured similar trials and tribulations.

During that fateful year, the dynamics between Lydia and me were…um…unique, due to our different backgrounds. As I've said, my economic background was comfortable. Lydia was a young woman from the inner city who was struggling to survive, as well as trying to make a better life for herself through education. We had divergent ideas and expectations of one another. I was raised to say "please" and "thank you" to everyone I met; Lydia, on the other hand, could not understand why I said these words to her because, after all, she was being paid to work for me. She even told me not to thank her because it was just a job, which she didn't like doing anyway! At that moment, I should have realized that these uneasy dynamics wouldn't produce a healthy relationship between us. As I'm sharing this with you, I can't remember specific examples, but I do recall our feelings of overall resentment.

Please bear in mind that Lydia was only the second PCA that I had ever had. I was neither educated enough at that time, nor was I seasoned enough to analyze and understand the multifaceted dynamics between a PCA and a person with a disability. In spite of this uncomfortable negativity, our professional relationship endured for a whole year, even though I was pretty much unaware of the abuse that was occurring. Lydia tried mightily to control me and abused me emotionally. She also stole money and credit cards from me. I remember one day I asked her, "Have you seen my sixty bucks? I thought I had it in my drawer, but now it's gone."

She replied, "Christine, you're so disorganized, I don't know where any of your shit is." She had a point there, but money and credit cards continued to disappear.

Out of that whole year of hell, the following story sticks out in my mind.

Lydia had not shown up for work for a week. I sorely needed her help with some household chores, especially laundry. It was very hard for me to do my laundry because the laundromat was at the top of a hill, and I lived at the bottom of that hill.

Of course, I ran out of underwear. Dammit to hell. I hate when that happens.

Let me digress with a bit of self-analysis. Sometimes I am a spoiled brat. It just so happens that the spoiled brat in me leaks out every so often, and this was one of those times. I awakened one morning and gloomily realized that I was down to my last pair of underpants. So I called Denise. (Denise and Lydia did not get along at all.) Denise was not too happy that I had called her at 8:30 in the morning.

"Denise, it's Chris."

There's a moment of silence, then:

"I know who you are because you call me every day, but I didn't think you would ever call me this early in the morning!" Remember, we had no cell phones, so when the phone rang, we answered it, hungover or whatever. P.S. Denise, my faithful friend, helped me with my underwear issue.

A week after the underwear incident, I decided to buy some happiness. I called a beautiful soul, someone special, and said, "My life is full of shit right now. So, New Year's Eve, let's have a kick-ass time! Wanna go away?"

She replied, "Absolutely! Let's go to Disney World." A few years earlier, for my high school graduation, my parents had given me a trip to Disney World, and my sister and I had had a great time. I was sure that my friend and I would have a rip-roaring New Year's Eve trip.

My New Year's Eves in the past had been nightmares. I figured maybe a trip would break the rotten luck that surrounded me on New Year's. Oh, how dead wrong I was. It was the trip from hell.

We arrived at Disney World on December 23 at 11:30 in the evening, and there was no one was in sight. The airport was barren. Normally, when I travel, there is a person waiting to assist my party and me to baggage claim. This time, I had rented a scooter because I felt that bringing my own scooter to the airport would be cumbersome. Since no one was there to help me, I had to walk to baggage claim with my walker at midnight. That was the kick-off for a vacation of misadventure. Neither my friend nor I were pleased about the lack of a scooter.

First of all, it was a major holiday. Can you imagine what those four days were like? We checked into our room that smelled like mildew. Due to the high occupancy of the Grand Floridian Hotel, there was no other room for us. I turned on the ceiling fan. Guess what? The freakin' fan didn't work, oh shit!

The next day, we decided to go to the Magic Kingdom. The park was packed and cold but we still had a great time. Fortunately, I found out something I had not known on my earlier Disney jaunt. It was the fact that when you use a scooter or a wheelchair, you can proceed to the front of the line for every ride. I noticed that people were taking advantage of this opportunity, unfortunately, just as people did with the accessible parking back at Ramapo. People who did not need wheelchairs were engaging in a façade. They were renting wheelchairs for the day, but it was obvious that they did not need them. I got over that deception in five minutes.

We had a wonderful day on The Pirates of the Caribbean, It's a Small World, The Log Flume, and so forth. The only ride I didn't like was Space Mountain because I couldn't see where the hell I was going. On the other hand, my friend loved, I mean really loved, Space Mountain. Later, I informed her that I had to use the bathroom. She told me that she'd wait for me in the store, and I should just look for her when I came out. I did what I had to do and went to look for my friend. She was nowhere to be found. Guess where she was? Well, I'll get to that later.

I started panicking. Someone had kidnapped her, but wait a minute, she was not a freakin' kid! I searched up and down Magic Kingdom in tears. I was thinking, "Maybe I can page her." There are no pagers in Magic Kingdom because everything's magical. An hour and a half later, guess who I saw approaching the gates? My friend–blithely smiling, singing, and dancing her way down USA Avenue. Meanwhile, I had been downing Prozac to calm my jittery nerves.

"Where the hell were you? I'm popping pills over you!"

"I was at Space Mountain, and there was no line! So I went on again and again and again. It was great!"

"No shit!" I didn't talk to her for two hours, but what made it worse was that she continued singing and smiling. Luckily, the next day, things went more smoothly. No major problems.

We decided to spend New Year's Eve in Epcot. We made reservations at the restaurant "Living under the Seas." We like seafood, however, we did not get seafood. We don't know what we got, but it wasn't seafood, I'll tell you that much. The after-dinner fireworks were taking place at midnight. We wanted to go on the popular ride, "Honey I Shrunk the Kids," but we also wanted to see the fireworks. Our plan was to see the fireworks and then run to that attraction. On the way to seeing the fireworks, my scooter began to act up. It kept stopping and starting. I knew what was happening. I hadn't plugged in the scooter to charge it the night before. No way was I gonna tell my friend the reality of the situation. But she, all-knowing, shouted, "What the hell is going on with that scooter?!"

I responded like a good little girl, "I don't know, but I think we need a plug."

"Christine, you didn't plug that in last night, did you?!"

"I don't know."

"Don't give me that bullshit!"

The end of the story was that we spent New Year's Eve in a museum nearby, the darkly lit India museum, with nonstop Indian music playing. I don't particularly care for Indian music, and neither does my friend, but that's where we found an electrical outlet.

Okay, so we each made our boo-boos, but when they say, "Leave the best for last," I have to agree. Especially regarding this Disney World sojourn. It was the last day of our rotten vacation. We decided to go to Universal Studios for half of the day and then catch a plane. Why didn't we think something would go wrong? I know why—wishful thinking. They say three is the magic number, and we had gotten three episodes out of the way. The fourth one was simply a bonus.

My friend and I ventured to the Earthquake ride, which was virtually empty. We hadn't expected to have our own attraction, but we did. Another big plus: No scooter hassles this time. The rules were that on some attractions, the attendants take the scooter to a different area, where the ride ends. That's unsettling because many of the young attendants don't really know how to operate the scooter. It always made me uneasy entrusting them with my invaluable "car keys" and "wheels." This time, however, the ride ended right where it began.

"Halle-freakin'-lujah! Nobody's gonna mess with my scooter! Yaay!"

By firmly holding both of my hands and forearms, my friend slowly guided me from my scooter into the ride's seat. Then the ride started, and it was a great one.

However, it was with some displeasure that we realized we couldn't see the attendant who had been watching my scooter. She also had the key. Where was she? Where was it? Finally, we spotted her and, mercifully, my scooter was safe and sound. My friend politely asked the attendant for my key. Her reply was, "Oh, don't worry; I gave it to another member in your party."

"What other member? We're a party of two! And we need that key!"

The woman was shocked. She had given the key to some man, who took it with a smile and placed it in his shirt pocket, as if it were a souvenir for the ride.

As I realized what was happening, I began to lose it. The scooter had been rented at Disney World, not Universal, and Universal couldn't do anything because the scooter was not their property. The attendant offered to look around the park a little, but she added nonchalantly, "I clock out in ten minutes."

After my friend argued with the manager for five minutes, she decided to look for the key holder herself. The manager was going to call the scooter company while she hunted throughout the park. Meanwhile I was left sitting on the scooter, keyless, and scared to death.

You might wonder why I was so terrified. I cannot walk without a walker. I had no walker, and no one could push the heavy scooter. I felt completely vulnerable, glued to the rotten scooter that wouldn't move.

Often I hear unknowing, able-bodied folks state that people with physical disabilities are "confined" to wheelchairs. But are they really confined if they can freely move about an architectural space? To the person with mobility issues, a scooter or a wheelchair is a device for freedom. I was confined this time because I could not jump out or roll out to catch my plane—with its take-off time looming nearer and nearer. I was helpless. Who enjoys that?

The helpful manager came back to inform me that he couldn't get in touch with the scooter company, and he didn't know what to do.

I replied, "I don't know what the hell to do, either!" Then he offered me a beverage; I replied, "Do you have a shot of tequila?" He just looked at me.

"What the hell would you do in my situation?" I demanded.

"I can get you a Diet Coke."

"I don't need a f'in' Diet Coke. Do you at least have a beer? And with a straw, please!!" I was loud and fuming.

That man was so terrified that he got me whatever I wanted. Later, after I had slurped down a couple beers, my friend reappeared and told me her bizarre story.

She had searched all over the park, with only a vague idea in her head as to the appearance of the family that been in front of us on the ride. After a wild pursuit, she at last found the family. "Do you have a key that a ride attendant gave you?"

Blank stares greeted her. "No—speak—English."

"Key, key, key!" In desperation she showed them one of her keys.

"Oh . . . key!" The dad fished the scooter key out of his shirt pocket, where he had placed it, believing it to be a free prize.

"Thank you." Then my friend ran back to me, where she found me downing beer and enjoying my situation. "You're tipsy! C'mon, we have a plane to catch."

After all…I made it back in one piece.

As I sit here writing, thinking about my life passages, the phone rings. Normally, I wouldn't even answer; however, Mac has been on my back lately about sprucing up our house and getting everything in tip-top order. In the past, I couldn't have cared less about that, but then my cousin, who is one month younger than I am, acquired a beautiful home—with beautiful kids. In addition to that unnerving event, I recently saw an exquisite model home that enhanced my motivation to fix up our own humble abode.

Dammit! Mac is always right. In his customary Zen manner, he told me, "We can move if you want to, Lucy." So last week I looked at homes, and this week, I'm remodeling our house, *instead* of moving because I (and Stevie) inherited from my grandfather the good old "iron wallet" (the cheap-as-hell lifestyle). We save lotsa money, but being frugal also means we get "red in the face."

The conversation between Mac and me progresses. I finally say "Okay, Mac. I guess we should remodel the house instead of buying a new one because I want that money to stay in the bank."

Next, I dutifully call the electrician, the painter, and the plumber. I also ask my dad if we should really spend money to redo the house. His reply is, "Mac's a great guy. He knows best. Listen to your husband for once."

Uh-oh, the phone is ringing again. Excuse me.

"Hello."

"Hello. This is Acme Chiropractor, calling to find out if you're interested in our current chiropractic wellness program."

"Yes, can you tell me more about it?"

"Uh—can—you—speak—Eng . . . lish? (They obviously didn't understand my speech.)

"Yes, and I was interested in your program, but since your attitude sucks, I am definitely *not* interested. Bye." Click. Some nerve.

The outstanding hero in life, my father, always told me that there are at least two sides to every story, and then there is the truth. My philosophy is the same as my father's. Now, dear reader, I realize that telemarketers need to make the greens; however, when someone is calling you at your house or at work, I think it's an invasion of personal space. Also, it intensifies when the telemarketer poses the question about my ability to speak English. I can understand that my accent can make it difficult for people to understand me *sometimes,* but it is still insulting when I am asked, "Are you sick? Can I call 911 for you?" or "Can I speak with your mommy or daddy?" It's not my job to always teach Disability Awareness when I'm out of the classroom, although I frequently do. Sometimes I just reply with my Jersey attitude, "No, but I can call 911 for your sorry f-in' ass!" Click.

Mac then says, "Lucy, that's not nice. You shouldn't say the 'F' word."

"Can I at least use 'ass'?"

"I think that word's nicer." What can I say? I like colorful language and I use it when I need to.

In 1994, I was twenty years old. Before then, my education had provided me with a door to my intimate relationships with others. A great benefit to my life, to be sure, but this did not directly start my career. Now, however, the groundwork for a career was being laid, even though I didn't know it. It amazes me how your initial career seems so separate from your personal stuff. As you venture into your work life, the personal aspect collides with the professional, and, hopefully, beautiful union results. But I'm getting too much ahead of myself.

The unconscious initial stages of my professional career had indeed started in 1994. The best way to describe this is symbolically. It began as a tiny, invisible puncture with a fixed circumference that opened more and more, finally revealing a whole picture of my future.

At that time, I had become an advocate for the disabled. The Leadership Conference for Students with Disabilities on University Campuses was preparing students for leadership roles on their respective campuses. Ms. Wexler recommended me to be a Peer Facilitator, which is an upperclassman serving as a co-instructor in the First Year Seminar course. So, I took a training course to become a Peer Facilitator. As Lydia was busy robbing and abusing me, I was a respected co-teacher/ Peer Facilitator for Dr. Harth. I fervently read the student journals and conducted various icebreakers. My feedback from students and Dr. Harth was outstanding. I felt very important.

Simultaneously, I experienced a rocky start to my public speaking career. If someone had said to me that I would one day become a professional public speaker and educator, a dedicated professor of Disability Studies, who would even write her memoirs, I would have bet a million dollars against it. And, today, I would be in debt for the rest of my freakin' life. This only serves to point out that the unexpected happens in life. Nevertheless, even back then, I knew I had tremendous compassion for people, especially students. Compassion has always been a great motivator for me.

Once I sat for hours in the dorm room of a student who had suicide ideation, and managed to persuade her to choose life. The Ramapo community was proud of me, but I'm not sharing this because I want you to think, "Oh, Christine, you're so wonderful." No, I'm sharing this with you because it was the first instance when I seriously considered "what I want to be when I grow up." But, of course, you never grow up because, hopefully, you never stop growing. And if you believe you're all grown up, then that would prove to me you have a lot of growing up to do. Simply put, I am glad and proud to be getting wiser and wiser every day.

Back to my first public speaking engagement. I didn't know what the hell I was doing. On my maiden voyage, I had a Diet Coke that I was sipping through a straw, and I suddenly burped mid-sentence in front of the class I was addressing. I was horrified. Never again! The second time after I spoke, I got a natural high from all the adrenaline pumping through my body. My public speaking career flowered. Who'd a-thunk it? Me, with my CP accent, an effective, provocative public speaker!

According to Erikson's theory of psychology, my psychosocial life development was right on track. Erikson states that when you are an adolescent (teenage years, to him, although I believe adolescence can extend into your early twenties), your main concern is yourself–me, me, me. Many individuals do not make it out of that "me" stage. Public speaking became my narcissistic "me" outlet. How so?

"Wow," I would say to myself. "I thrill so many people. I'm fabulous! People love to hear me speak. I'm just terrific!" And that was okay at that point of my life; it was an appropriate time for my self-affirmation due to the difficulties I had been through.

I was asked to speak at quite a few engagements at Ramapo. I was an inspiration for everyone on campus. I continued to think that I was "The Bomb" and "The Shit," meaning I was awesome. But I also had a reality meter. After a speaking engagement, I would scooter alone back to my home. In my apartment, which had started to look teenier and teenier, I tried to keep the glow going, sometimes successfully, sometimes not. I pretty much lived only for the moment, whether good or bad, and I was entirely ignorant of the blossoming, long-term transition from negative to positive self-esteem. I was incapable of realizing the enormity of what was happening inside me.

So after wowing my audience, I landed back at home. I went inside to face an "audience" that was surely the polar opposite of the public speaking crowd. Lydia was there, and I turned back into a frail, terrified soul, afraid for my life.

I believe Lydia was emotionally and mentally abusive. Consequently I have repressed ninety-five percent of my memories about her. All I can remember was talking about her to Fred and Denise, who were prime witnesses to my "torture." I was extremely narcissistic concerning my public speaking, and narcissistic being Lydia's employer, abuse notwithstanding. It's easy to understand narcissism when you get lots of applause, but if you're confused as to how I was narcissistic concerning Lydia, let me explain.

I didn't believe that she would keep my confidentiality. Actually, I thought if I fired her, she would ruin my life. Everything was all about me. I lived in fear that she would tell my parents all about my friends and the times that I enjoyed so much with Fred. I was afraid that she would hurt me physically. As I think about it now, she was *looking* to get fired, but my narcissism got the best of me—resulting in my not firing her because *everything* was all about me!

The summer before my senior year at Ramapo consisted of my secretly dating Fred and steadfastly keeping it secret from my parents. I realized then that I was not in love with Fred. Our paths were heading in diverging directions. I gave up on love, and I almost gave up on education, as well. Lydia had graduated that May, and much to my chagrin, I was looking for a new PCA despite the fact that I had never fired Lydia. I didn't move back home with my parents that summer, and Ramapo agreed that I could stay in my wonderful apartment, if I took a required course, Statistics, which was worth three credits. Although I love math because it's like solving a puzzle, my math course that summer was not high on my list of priorities.

Pat and Ann Chang and I were the only people in the main building at Ramapo. At times, that was kinda creepy, so you may wonder why I wanted to stay there, rather than be home with my parents. I did because the campus *was* my community, and for better or worse, my apartment was my home. I desperately wanted to be independent. More important, the apartment was accessible to suit my needs. The house in which I grew up was not accessible, except for my room and bathroom. My heavenly apartment was so small that the microwave, refrigerator, and sink were easily within my reach and thereby provided me the freedom to eat by myself. Believe me, that's a cherished freedom. In truth, I had moved out of my parents' sumptuous home when I started my life as a college woman. And I didn't move back in, except for the relatively short period of time when my current townhouse was being built.

During the fall of my senior year at Ramapo, I had the honor of co-teaching my first course. The respected Dr. Chang was the professor. I was his Peer Facilitator. I'm fortunate that he keeps reappearing in my life. He has always believed in me. He gave me the opportunity to co-teach, and I shared *full* teaching responsibilities with him. To this very day, Pat Chang and Mike Fluhr have been the two most influential mentors in my life. In my experience, having a good mentor is more important than having good grades. Don't get me wrong, grades are important, and not all mentors impart their internal values, but a good mentor teaches you all about people skills. That is the key to success. Networking is the golden ticket.

In my current teaching capacity, I tend to analyze the students I'm educating. In this regard, the Internet has its plusses and minuses. The plusses are that students can type faster than I can talk. They can get research online, and a ten-page paper for them is equivalent to a five-page paper written less than a decade ago. I know if my students are reading this, they're flipping out! They'll see themselves in my story, about how most professors still require a research paper. I do, in every class. So, last semester, I was grading papers when I noticed in one that the fonts were all different colors. The student had copied and pasted research and had not bothered to change the color. Another crafty pupil cited a website that I know he hadn't utilized. Students tend to type away, navigating the Web so they can come up with a ten-page paper in only a day. Some of these papers are good, and some are lousy. But none of the students did it the way I did it. The good old-fashioned way was to sneak a sandwich into the library because my butt was going to be planted there all day, doing research. And my butt *was* planted there all day, day after day, sneaking in that sandwich, which I ate in the library bathroom because it was too cold to go outside.

I became wiser about how to use the library through my friendship with the librarian, Kevin. He obtained the requested journals and books and brought them out to us fledgling researchers. I had to fill out an itty-bitty tiny freakin' piece of paper requesting my materials. And Kevin would take my teensy tidbit of a paper, go back into book storage, and deliver the sacred book to me, if I was lucky. If I was not lucky, I got the damn microfiche. And that was really a bitch, let me tell you. Microfiche was one of the mandated sources for a research paper at that time. My CP coordination intensified the anger I felt for the entire microfiche-addicted academic world as I attempted to thread the toilet paper-shaped roll through the machine. When I got to the page I wanted, I was damn lucky if I didn't see a big blotch on the film where I needed the info.

Today, Kevin the librarian sits in front of a computer, where we share many a meaningful conversation. I'm so glad he has a new office, removed from the Ramapo student body. On a weekly basis, I go in and say to him, "These freakin' students are so lazy!!! And I haven't gotten laid in a week!"

He replies, "That's all you got to complain about? Go home."

We bullshit for a while and I go home.

As I said, that autumn was my first real experience co-teaching. Pat Chang was the most amazing teacher that anyone could want. It was a delight being his Peer Facilitator and I still use his gems of wisdom with my students. We had a class that was unique unto itself. When a professor creates an environment where students feel comfortable and safe, personalities tend to flourish for the duration of that class. And boy, we had some personalities.

At the end of every class, we had a one-minute paper that was written anonymously as a reaction to that particular class. Pat typed them up, and did we have some discussions about those papers. He even took his class camping on the Ramapo Indian Reservation, a mile from campus, in weather that was 20 degrees Fahrenheit. I tried, but I chickened out. I went to the reservation, but it was unbearably cold. Pat said, "Go home." That was hard to do. I felt I owed it to my students to stay, but I followed his sage advice. At a frigid two o'clock in the morning, I returned to my apartment.

That weekend, I decided to visit my parents in lieu of the camping trip. When I arrived, I was excited to receive some kind of an invitation in the mail. Who had sent it? Oh, wow, it was a wedding invitation from Rick. You know, Rick with the freakin' paddle. Rick and I had been pretty close the summer before. He was completing a final course at Ramapo, and he asked if he could room with me on campus. I said, "Sure." Everyone thought we were getting it on, but I swear I never touched that man. We slept in separate beds and talked about relationships, like why I was with Fred, because everyone knew I did not love him and that included Fred. Rick was wrestling with the same issue about why he was with Denise. He really, really loved her, but they had problems. So what? Every couple has problems.

But you don't know the big freakin' monumental issue here. When I first saw Rick's wedding invitation, I had to read the damn thing ten times because *Denise's* name wasn't on the invitation. He was marrying some other chick he'd knocked up during a cataclysmic one-night stand. Amazingly, ten years later, they are still happily married with four beautiful kids.

As I'm writing this, I miss the friendships that have swirled in and out of my past. Dear friends are of the utmost importance to me. In these memoirs, the topic of "best friends" has been steadily present in my heart. For me, that "best friend" relationship is sometimes ephemeral. The question is, *who* will linger? Is length of relationship a crucial criterion for treasured friendship? I think we say too often and too easily, "so and so is my best friend," especially in high school and college. I've certainly done that in the past and sometimes still do. Who really is someone's best friend? What are the essential factors in friendship? Are you your only best friend? Given the zigs and zags and the metaphorical staircase of oppression in my life, are best friends short-lived or are they rock solid? Do they metamorphose over time?

Most of my best friendships seem eternal, but not all. Mac says that I'm his best friend, but he's not really mine, although it often feels that way. He's my husband. He's my co-provider, my confidant, my just-about-everything, but not my best friend. Reflecting on my life, I don't have a best friend at this time. Wisdom and insight have brought me to this conclusion. With all my "honor roll" accomplishments, I have un-met friendship expectations and that includes friendship with myself.

Now, I bet you're saying, "Isn't she contradicting herself regarding best friends, past and present?" Good. Don't be afraid to ask questions. Relax, listen up, and ponder how my "best friend" philosophy might apply to your life situation, as people enter and exit your life. Yes, I'm contradicting myself. I'll probably contradict myself on other musings about friendship, and frankly, on just about any thoughtful topic. That's my nature, a bunch of human ironies.

I'll ramble on because this topic has to do with the meaning of life, at least for me. I think friendships are represented symbolically by lovely eddies of leaves, swirling in and out of one's life. Ideally, the treasure of various friendships leaves an indelible print behind. This weaves the tapestry of our lives. It is essential, ever changing, present and not present, but present in our hearts. Those "best friend" relationships have always been dependent on what was transpiring at any given time. In that respect, this also defines my relationship with my mom. My mom has always been there for me. I am so fortunate. Many women have far less.

Meanwhile, back at the ranch. I had given up on love. You know, that intimacy in a relationship. Fred was just around to be around. A good buddy, I guess. So there you have it: I gave up on love, and for a short time, I gave up on my education. "Damn it to hell" was my theme song.

"Now why should I bust my ass in school, if I have a trust fund?" I asked myself. Not a big trust fund, but I was comfortable. I guess the answer was and remains that I want to prove to the non-disabled world that I am non-disabled, too. No, wait, hold on there—that's not really it. I have Disability Pride. I just want genuine equality of opportunity. Who doesn't?

During my last semester at Ramapo, I had suicide ideation. I got a lot of help at that time, especially concerning how to understand my parents. Friends held onto me. And I thank them for saving my life.

I try to live a relatively humble life, just like my father. I have always liked living humbly, below my means. But at the end of my senior year, my parents, especially my mother, had plans for me. I informed my parents that I would not be moving back with them. They were horrified. I informed them that I wanted to rent an apartment in Plainfield, which was $400 a month, in an urban setting "on the other side of the tracks." Boy, would I stick out like a sore thumb—a young, white chick on a scooter, bouncing around the largely African American community. Sounded super cool to me. Hot damn! After weeks of silence, my parents announced that it would be best if I could move into a condo with attached garage. All my own; modern, and completely accessible. I flipped out because of all the g's I had to put up.

Life in my itsy-bitsy abode, with the haunted bed and the vintage 1969 refrigerator, came to an end over a two-month period. During those last couple months, I was searching frantically for the type of condo my parents wanted, one with an attached garage and a master bedroom with an accessible bathroom. My search was arduous. Those Plainfield apartments were looking better and better. I distinctly remember coming home on the weekends just to canvass the Union County edition of *The Star Ledger*. I would scour the listings for condos, townhouses, and regular houses. Nowadays, I would have just stayed in my little apartment and searched on the Internet. The good thing was that I was able to spend time with my interesting family.

Then my dad found the perfect condo accidentally. He owns a company that installs windows for commercial buildings and he and my mom are quite accustomed to working on Sundays. My mom sits in the car, while my dad goes into every building and inspects his workers' progress. As a youngster I always knew my mother's feelings about the work because I was in the car right beside her.

So on this particular Sunday afternoon my father discovered this elegant townhouse complex. Not surprisingly, he snuck into a townhouse under construction. He came striding out, declaring, "Teresa, this is perfect for Christine."

I think my mother wanted to kill him at that point, but it was absolutely perfect, a dream come true.

They drove home and Dad called me at my apartment to inform me of his terrific discovery. It sounded like everything I wanted in a condo, even though the town was a little too white and a little too snobby for me, but I said "Oh well." The next day, Dad and I went to the office where they had the models. We walked in and announced, "We want to purchase the model with the master bedroom on the first floor." The gentleman informed us that there were no more models left, and that there was a waiting list, and that you could not even get on the waiting list. Just my luck.

"Shit, I'm gonna live with my parents for the rest of my damn life." (As I've said before, the spoiled brat in me comes out from time to time.)

"Dad, I really, really want to live here. It's perfect. It's everything I need, and more. I'm disabled—can't we use that?!" I was fishing here. I really wanted the place.

During that summer when I visited my parents, I would drive up to Zen Farms (as I called it) and just cry. I glumly gave up on my dream house and returned to my tiny dive in Ramapo. I was in the midst of packing in the front room when my bathroom phone rang. It was a hot summer day, and, of course, the 1969 air conditioner was taking a vacation. I don't know how, but I managed to answer the phone in time, which I rarely ever do, due to my CP.

"Dad, who died?" My dad only calls me if it's a tragic moment, or if I got in trouble and he found out.

"Chris, no one died."

"Oh, shit, what did I do now?" I asked myself.

"You got the townhouse!"

"Get the hell outta here, oops, I mean heck. Sorry, Dad. Great! How the hell did that happen?"

Dad told me, and again I am reminded that networking is the key. It is whom you know, and this is a prime example. Remember in my childhood years when I double-dated with my dad, Kelly, and her daddy? Well, Kelly's daddy was a very influential man. It just so happened that a very good friend of his was the owner of the building company that was managing the project. They built an additional model *just for me.* How spoiled can you get? Charlie kept on saying, "You don't want that damn condo; you'll have to drive up and down Route 22." That was one helluva busy highway. But I didn't care—I love to drive fearlessly on highways and parkways. And after I finally got the condo, Charlie was thrilled.

While my condo was under construction, I was filled with anticipation. It was like a dream come true. Not only would I have my own place, I'd have my own completely *accessible* place. The only problem was that it would take a year to build. I was moving out of my apartment and had nowhere to go. So where do you think I went? Back to my parents and their inaccessible house. My mom was overjoyed. I think she subconsciously believed the condo would never be completed, and if it was, I would back out, and her little girl would stay with her forever. Oh, she was so wrong.

Moving back to my parents' house wasn't that bad. I was doing my senior internship at Kessler Institute and vigorously planning my strategy to move into an interim apartment. Unfortunately, that never happened. You win some, you lose some.

Everything was moving along smoothly. Kessler was going okay, and I'll share more interesting details on my career there after the following story, which had a huge impact on me.

Recently (about ten years after these events), I had a conversation with my mother over morning coffee.

I asked, "Was it hard for you to let me go?"

"Of course, but you were so determined that nothing was going to hold you back. From the beginning, we've been proud of you for that. And by the time you were twenty-four, you were your own woman. A parent couldn't ask for more."

"Would you have ever kicked me out?"

"Never. Life was hard for you, Christine, and it still is. As a mother, although I remain enormously proud of you, it broke my heart to see my disabled daughter alone in her own place. I wanted to take care of you forever, but obviously you had alternative plans. And you were right."

It's not often that a parent tells her adult child they are right and the parent is in error. Plus, considering the monumental nature of my moving out, my mom exhibited extraordinary faith in me and was unabashed to admit her mistake in judgment. On her part, that demonstrated humility, honesty, and unconditional love. Most people cannot say this about a parent, and I can truthfully say it about both my parents. I'm very lucky in that respect.

Near the beginning of my memoirs, as you may recall, I talked about several disability identification models. My mom was a prime example of the Moral Model because she wanted very much to take dutiful, loving care of her heaven-sent angel. Who can blame her? When I was very young, she could never envision that I would be a productive, independent woman. She is partially right because life is extremely challenging, difficult, and exhausting every single day when you have a major physical disability. CP, which affects the way I walk, talk, eat, and the way I breathe, particularly at night, is especially challenging. My personal question in life is: How did my super-busy, hungry, questioning mind get hooked up with this body? I'm always ready for the next adventure, but my body and stamina give out, and I'm forced to rest and recuperate at home for a day or two. Yeah, right, that lousy word "rest." Lousy, because I'm forced to rest against my will. My body needs rest and relaxation, due to my respiratory condition. Also, my muscles ache, and spasticity intensifies the pain. This is my reality. And I still appreciate the faith my parents demonstrated in me from the beginning.

This morning as Mac is applying make-up on me (what a guy!), he says with concern that the dark rings around my eyes are getting bigger and bigger. True. My soul has more energy than the average person. I cannot even sit and enjoy a movie by myself. My mother has always been energetic, too. I never saw *her* sit and watch TV. So if I'm sitting, watching TV, I equate it with being a lazy bum. People are sometimes amazed at my academic and professional accomplishments at the age of thirty-something. In reality, I wish my accomplishments had come more slowly and steadily over a longer period of time. I don't take the time for little oases of peace and tranquility; instead, I charge headlong into the next item of business. Hence, the dark circles under my tired eyes.

Mac has taught me to enjoy life more and to joyously embrace our cultural differences, as well as our different identity models. (There are more than the ones I have discussed, so far. Just read on to understand.) Recently Mac and I discovered a town in New Jersey that we both like because of the scenic drive there and its lovely, quaint houses and restaurants. It just so happens that this quaint community with its quaint scenery has little black lawn jockeys on all the front lawns. Is this the northern version of the KKK? My beautiful black Zen husband strolls along the streets and kisses my white face when we go into a store. At first, I could not understand why he would want to come back to this beautiful, seemingly bigoted town. He states, "If I stay out of town, they win. What's the point in that, Lucy? No one is going to force me out of no f-in' town." I believe that with his calm and polite manner, he is changing their point of view. That is noteworthy. Plus, he means it–he very rarely uses the f-word and a double negative at the same time!

Back to the point of Mac showing me the good life. That's true; however, as a Buddhist, he doesn't lack what I lack: calmly living and enjoying the world at large and all that is in it. (Yes, my Zen husband and I are always furiously on the go.) He has a more balanced attitude about the rush of life. He is so tolerant and patient with the world. What a guy.

As I see the Ramapo students run to class, I am amazed yet again that probably sixty percent of them did not get any sleep last night and are attending class drunk and high. As I let down my ramp, I hear, "Professor McCohnell! What did I miss last week?" Shit, it's before twelve noon, and I haven't finished my Starbucks. How the hell am I supposed to know what she missed? This is typical of the questions I get in my professional career!

"Umm, uh, I'm running late. I'll email you, or better yet, I won't! Email Rose. She was in class last week." If I were to email every student who asked, "What did I miss last week?" I would still be at Ramapo and never, ever have left for the weekend.

As of September 2007, I was in my fifth year of teaching at Ramapo. In the beginning, I didn't know what I was doing. Now I know some secrets that make my life a hell of a lot easier. For example, I include a statement in my syllabus that addresses "What did I miss last week?" That's why I have the students work in groups. If you miss something, ask your group members. This arrangement is best for all of us.

"Okay, Professor McCohnell. See ya tonight."

As I walk to the A-wing, I notice, in the corner of my eye, the colorful leaves of autumn ever so delicately blowing in the wind. Ah, a Zen image of my many thoughts on friendship. A friend is like a colorful leaf, in my thinking. Family is the trunk of the tree; it's the base. It never goes away. Did you ever hear someone say, "She would never be my friend, *but she is family*"? Like friends, the leaves fall off the tree. But the trunk is permanent. Just like family . . .oh, yeah, family; excuse me, I was daydreaming again.

My latest self-discovery is that I finally understood that when my family life is in chaos, I work myself super-duper hard and never take breaks. Damn! What am I saying? I married someone who makes me enjoy life. *Mac is my immediate family now,* not my siblings and parents. I am free from that habit of chaos due to the peaceful environment Mac and I have created.

The famous Kessler Institute and I first united more than a decade ago. My senior fieldwork was in the Education Department at Kessler in West Orange, New Jersey. I immersed myself in attempting to create Disability Awareness programs. In creating my programs, I discovered that non-disabled folks exhibited limited, surface esteem in regard to disability awareness. It makes sense, right? Everyone wants to feel the type of "high" I had after speaking at Ramapo, seeing myself as an inspirational Super Crip and an admired poster-child-of-sorts . . . helping the less fortunate crips while appealing to the non-disabled masses. Yes, indeed, appealing to the non-disabled masses. You know, like the cure-seeking telethon bit and that antiquated patriarchal thinking, primarily focusing on curing poor, sweet, angelic children and not focusing on the far-less cute adults, who have grown up with Multiple Sclerosis (or any disability). In fact, a number of these former poster children of telethons gone by, who are now grown-up activists and virtually forgotten, call themselves "Jerry's Orphans."

Most non-disabled folks want to *medically eliminate* the important disability culture by *curing* the disability, rather than working toward complete social inclusion in all walks of life. An inclusive country (or world) would insure that *all* banks, doctors' offices, restrooms, restaurants, subways, taxis, reception halls, museums, schools, universities, theatres, delis, busses, and so on, were completely accessible.

In *Why I Burned My Book,* famed disability historian Paul Longmore says that looks are deceiving. For example, a ramp is not enough. A ramp is certainly a *visible* disability accommodation, but it's just a beginning. We also need doors that are at least thirty-six inches wide. Those doors must be easy to open, and not so heavy that folks with limited strength in their upper bodies can't open the damn doors unless they're automatic. Talking elevators with Braille, as well as large print, Braille, and picture symbols on menus, signs, and, well—everywhere! Recognition that service animals are not pets, and, as a result, these service animals must be allowed everywhere—not just as *stated* in the current laws, but in reality. Universal design in all new buildings—which benefits everyone! Sign language, especially for all political discussions and debates, as well as snappy primetime TV shows.

We, as a nation, could use more than a little info on disability *pride.* Pride? Yes, pride. Such a revamped society does not fit the overriding Moral and Medical models of cure-all, eradicate-the-problem telethons. Nowadays a good number of middle-aged couples (specifically U.S. citizens) that are expecting a baby willingly undergo *in utero* genetic testing. Sounds practical, but an untold number of these would-be parents terminate fetuses with disabilities like Down syndrome, spina bifida, or others detected *in utero.* Disability is usually disparaged and not considered a source of pride and inclusion. That must change, also.

Ah, eliminating disability, rather than including it. And it's all so easy because we generally have society's applause and blessing. Just make disability disappear rather than change our attitudes about it. Sounds great, right? Sounds a bit Hitleresque to me. Did you know that an integral part of Hitler's Final Solution was murdering multitudes of people with disabilities, as well as brutally experimenting on them, no matter what their ethnicity or religion? In other words, the Nazis also tried to eradicate disability, which essentially, would have eradicated me—and other people with disabilities.

Did you know that in the early twentieth century when masses of immigrants arrived at Ellis Island, people with disabilities were sent back home? One test of ability included walking up the many steps at Ellis Island. If you couldn't walk up the steps, good-bye. Give me your tired, your poor, but keep your damn disabled.

The unspoken motto is "Cure 'em or kill 'em." Or simply institutionalize 'em. Or don't hire 'em. The grossly disproportionate unemployment rate for persons with disabilities is a whopping eighty-six percent! Now that's discrimination.

Well, guess what? People with disabilities don't always want to be "cured" or be an inspiration for the masses. We just want to be normal citizens—because, after all, disability *is* normal.

Don't get me wrong, everyone, including me, wants to see a cure for AIDS and cancer and more. I'm talking about healthy people with disabilities, not unlike me, who are not interested in a cure for their disability. Believe it or not, there are lots of people in wheelchairs and scooters who feel this way. This kind of disability pride is quite strong in the Deaf community and elsewhere. In fact, the word "cure" is not completely absent from the voices of Disability Rights activists. Many of us simply wish that "cure," in the sense of eradication of the so-called problem, not be the primary focus. Attitudes need to change.

There are fifty-four million people in the USA right now (2008) who have disabilities. Did you know that the vast majority of those disabilities are *acquired* during a lifetime and not genetically transmitted? About eighty percent of all American citizens will acquire a disability, or have a close loved one acquire a disability, in a lifetime.

Well, I'm getting a little off track here, although the digression was important. But I'll fill you in on something big at this juncture. Again, my life is a paradox. Although I have been talking about my past, I currently strongly desire a cure for a most beloved family member. My knight in shining armor, my precious, wonderful brother Stevie, has just been diagnosed with brain cancer. I am filled with enormous sorrow. Everything seems ugly and futile. Sobbing helps, and it doesn't help. I can't even write about it now. Please, God—whoever you are, help me. I need the strength.

The paradox of existence. The here and the hereafter, whatever they are.

Returning to the renowned Kessler Institute…

There was a decided absence of people with disabilities in the Education Department at Kessler, and this struck me as well beyond odd. Why? Partly because many people even *with* disabilities are clueless about the rich history of the Disability Rights Movement, identification models, and Disability Culture. I realized at that time that I did not know of any curriculum for Disability Studies. Right then and there, I decided to (1) create just such a needed and informative curriculum, (2) diligently get to work teaching said curriculum, and (3) abandon my "Super Crip inspiration" mentality.

Fred and I were, as usual, on and off. As I've asked, you know how you love someone, but you're not in love with him? No doubt about it, Fred was in love with me, and I loved him as a friend "with benefits." Sad to say, I continued to keep Fred a secret. I realized that our lives were going in different directions. The Seton Hall Masters Program really separated us. My ambitions and my associations with high-achiever personalities didn't connect with my relaxed, carefree, laid-back time with Fred.

I sometimes wonder how I ended up with a calm Zen-follower like Mac. I have already said that a person like Mac can be calm and subdued, as well as being a high achiever. I believe that my husband is the next Dalai Lama--with the energy of a three-year-old. Okay, that's an exaggeration, but you get the picture. Unlike Fred, Mac wants to achieve so much. On his days off from work, he's just as active as a little kid. In that way, Mac and I are similar. But as I get older, although I am a high achiever, I often want to be relaxing at home, while Mac always wants to explore new things, go out on weekends, and just get busy enjoying life. I hope you can see that a high achiever who is occasionally subdued (me), combined with a calm person who is also a very high achiever and never wants to stay at home (Mac), can enjoy a solid relationship and attain serenity. Indeed, such a combination can produce a great union. Have you ever experienced that?

As I'm writing this, I'm wondering if Mac is going to divorce me after reading my memoirs. I can always lie and say, "I totally made things up to make my book a titillating bestseller!" And I bet he would look at me serenely and reply, "Whatever you say, Lucy." His self-confidence is sexy.

All right, enough of that. Onto my past faults, frailties, and sins: Here's one of my best good old-fashioned juicy stories.

My friend Ann and I decided to go to Rochester, New York at the last minute to attend a disability conference. Two years prior to that, I had attended the same conference with my mother. I had had a really good time before, and Ann wanted to get away for the weekend. Since she was a Special Ed teacher, this conference would fulfill multiple purposes. As I think about it, I laugh at how it all turned out.

Attending that second conference had a huge impact on my life. An intense love affair started there. As I've stated before, I have kissed with many men in my life—in fact, too many. Deep in my soul, I know I have morals. I had intercourse with only three guys before my husband. I think I might have told you that already, but it bears repeating. Why? Because each guy I slept with, I still have feelings for. Matt was one of them.

Ann and I took the long drive up to Rochester. Ann's wedding was going to be in a couple of months, and I was contemplating disclosing to my parents my relationship with Fred. The subject of men consumed our six-hour conversation-drive. The first night, we attended a dance performance. During that performance, I was so impressed by the wheelchair dance; a ballet performed by a wheelchair artist named Matt and his non-disabled partner. I said to Ann, "This is amazing. And he's so hot! Why are all the good men married?" I assumed he was married to his Cinderella-like dance partner, which was the general buzz.

Ann replied, "All I got to say is, do you really want to be with Fred?"

"Yes, um, I'm not exactly sure, but I don't think so."

Fred would soon be a footnote from the past.

Ann turned in early at 10 o'clock. I usually went to bed at ten, too, but I couldn't sleep, so, what did I do? I went to the bar! On the way there, I discovered that Matt was not married. I passed him in the hallway as he was entering another woman's room--*not his partner's room.* And I'm not gonna lie--I was ecstatic! Remember that I liked "players," and I figured that he was one.

A year later, I found out that Matt had never, ever been a player, and I broke his heart. His heart was broken, and my heart was shattered. Anyway, back to the story.

The next day, I was alone, scootering along, minding my own business. Suddenly, out of the blue someone called loudly, "Hey you, what's your name?"

My smart-ass self replied, "I know you're not talking to me, asshole." I thought, "Who the hell does he think he is just barking out like that?"

He replied, "You have an attitude problem."

I replied, "You don't talk to people like that, by yelling at them, asshole!"

I guess we clicked. After conversing for a half hour, he provided me with the proverbial phone number and screen name. God, he was sexy, intelligent, and cocky. He was from Puerto Rico and had long black hair. His body was incredible. On the way home, Ann and I resumed our conversation. When she and I finally reached my townhouse, I had decided to pursue Matt. The whole drive all I had thought about was sleeping with that man. Fred was less and less my sexual desire, and I soon told him so.

Matt and I had online conversations for hours on end. Online conversations led to phone conversations. Being "in love" is tricky. Can you be in love for eight months at a distance, or is that considered mere infatuation? I don't know, but that's how it was. And it was something!

Soon thereafter, I decided to pack my bags and stay with him. It was one of the best times in my life. We clicked emotionally and physically. His family thought I was wonderful, and I felt the same about them. However, my parents were pissed at me, to say the least, and Fred was concerned. But I was having the time of my life. It was the honeymoon of all honeymoons! As I watched him dance, I wanted him more. We were crazy about each other, but artists tend to be more than a wee bit self-centered, and that was Matt's problem. I started to miss my home. I actually wanted to return to that now-hostile environment.

For that week, we shared a little apartment. Niagara Falls was our place. We had our songs, and it was perfect. The day I left, I had a feeling that I would never see him again. And sadly enough, that was the truth. We continued our phone conversations, and I wanted him to move down to my townhouse. He was so old-fashioned that he believed he needed a job and lots of money to support me. Years later, we both believed that we had made a mistake by giving up on our relationship. Out of all the men in my life, Matt filled me with the most fiery passion and what I assumed would be a lifelong, romantic connection. Our opposite situations attracted. I was an academic Jersey woman, and he was my singing man. He told me that he had never sung for another woman.

We communicated for a month online, when I was preparing to get married. He asked me to stop the wedding. Instant gratification, yes, but not the genuine, long-term relationship I yearned for. Real love is peaceful. And the families must be considered. Matt and I would never have lasted. We were too argumentative and high strung with one another. He also had a serious drinking problem, and God knows I didn't want to invite more alcoholism into my circle. But he'll always be my singing man.

My education took a back seat that summer while I was upstate. But I still cared about it, so that fall I was back to attending a Masters program at Seton Hall University. Upon graduation from Ramapo, the last thing I had wanted to do was to go back to school. I declared I did not need or want my Master's degree. I was no different than many twenty-one-year-olds; I thought I knew everything. I bet you can probably relate to that. For a time, I even joined Matt's dance troupe as a semi-pro.

I'm now gonna whisk you back *before* that fateful second Rochester conference. After first leaving Ramapo, I had decided to start my own motivational speaking company called Empowerment, which I soon incorporated. Of course, I thought my business was going to be magnificent. I obtained all the media items that one needs to market an emerging company. I had a selling line. I created business cards. A motivational speaking company communicating to and about the disability community on a factual level! I thought I was gonna hit it big. Come to find out, if you don't have experience or a Master's, your company will go under in six months. Empowerment went under within a year. (Later, when I met Matt, he wrote his phone and address on one of my business cards because he did not have anything else he could write on. I still have that card.)

After realizing that Empowerment was surely dying, I had a conversation with my treasured mentor, Pat Chang. What should I do now? He encouraged me to go to for my Master's degree. I replied, "Hell, no!"

"Just fill out the application, take the GRE exam, and I'll write you a kick ass recommendation."

I applied to only one school, hoping I would not get in. Earlier that year, I had gone to Seton Hall to visit my friend, Sandy. So I decided to apply to Seton Hall, what the hell. That's how I decided on a school.

I took the GRE and did poorly, just like my SATs, so I was sure I would be declined by their Master's Program in Counseling. Pat *must* have written a kickass recommendation as promised because I was accepted with open arms. Well, I *had* done very well academically in acquiring my Bachelor's degree. All that hard undergraduate work had paid off. Well, kind of. At first, I hadn't wanted to go to *any* college, let alone Seton Hall.

I will never, ever forget the day I discovered that I had been accepted into the program. Kim and I had gone to Bridgewater Mall to see the movie "The Truman Show" with Jim Carrey. When we got home I "ran" into the house to use the bathroom. Meanwhile, my sister was looking through the mail. She yelled out from the kitchen, "You got something from Seton Hall!"

"Is it small? 'Cuz if it's small, it's a rejection letter. Open it up." A few seconds later I asked, "So where are we eating tonight?"

She answered, "You might want to read this."

She opened the door and handed me my acceptance letter. I can tell my step-grandchildren that I was accepted into the Seton Hall Master's Program in Counseling while I was on the bowl. Now that's something! I called my parents and we were all overjoyed at this new adventure in my life.

At the same time that I adopted an egotistic attitude due to getting into the Master's Program, I worked on Empowerment, which was fast dying. I kept hoping against hope that it would prosper. While my professional career was going down the tubes, my personal life sucked, as well. Then, my cherished buddy, one of the true loves of my life, was getting married again. Stevie, my older brother had gotten a divorce and we had regained time for our relationship. We'd even gone to Club Med together, like old times. We had so much fun,. That pissed me off. He even brazenly invited the new girl out to dinner with us! What can I say? Again, I was really, really pissed. Actually, that week was and was not a great one.

Later on, as then-faithful Stevie and Mary were planning their wedding, my selfish streak got to me. Either I was angry because he was getting married or because Mary had decided to have the reception upstairs, with no elevator. I was in the wedding party. We had long velvet dresses for the crisp November weather. It was a huge bridal party, and the special thing about it was that all the attendants were siblings of the bride and groom. I thought that was endearing. It was just immediate family, and that touched my heart. As for my angrily "walking" up the stairs, I had been too narcissistic to remember that it was Mary's day.

During the happy wedding, my mother didn't feel well at all. We found out that she had Bell's palsy and couldn't drive. She had Bell's palsy for three months. Kim and I drove her everywhere. Kim would do absolutely anything for our parents.

I clearly remember that Christmas. My mom still had Christmas for us, even though she could not see out of one eye because of her diabetes. She had a little Christmas tree that my dad had bought for her. While preparing the festivities, my mother spilled some gravy on the floor, with forty-five people soon coming over. Only my sister and Aunt Barb helped. I tried to help, but wasn't successful--I think I broke a dish or two.

I spent most of my time brooding. Everyone was living outside the house except me. Shit! But I had a hunch that everything would be worth the wait, and I was right. My new home, my condo, turned out to be perfect. All the bullshit I had had to go through to get the damn place completely disappeared from my consciousness. As you might recall, my father's friend had connections so that I could have the exact model I wanted in Zen Farms. They built a model just for me, which was incredible, but the driveway was so steep that my father was unhappy. I was crushed because I had really wanted that particular model, Number 25, due to its location nestled off the street.

My father often says, "Have I ever given you a bum steer in life?" That's his famous quote. I have to admit it--my father has never, ever given me a bum steer. Maybe I'm still waiting for that to happen. Unlikely. We decided I should move into 69 Harmony Way instead. That townhouse could be fairly easily modified to be accessible. Plus, the garage, double car park, and gently sloping driveway were perfect. The new residence was officially mine! Mom was "head decorator," even though we had a professional, and I selected every fabric and color. It was Paradise.

The neighborhood was reputed to have haunted spirits abiding there. Spirits who have supposedly dwelled and spooked there since dying in the Revolutionary War. Happily, they have never physically appeared. Also happily, to this day, no person ever wants to leave my charming townhouse, once they've entered. Why? It's well organized and very comfy and homey. I don't know if there's magic in this house, or if a good bunch of quiet overseeing spirits actually do live here with me. In addition to the neighborhood having survived the Revolutionary War, my townhouse property had been an old farm once upon a time. Maybe those hearty, earthy spirits from the past still live here, after all. Frankly, I welcome the unorthodox company. That's the way I like it.

Back to *my* past:

We put an automatic door from the garage into the house so I just push a button, and magically, the door opens. My dad, with his genius in construction, was able to design an accessible bathroom. There was only one other minor change, but it definitely made a world of difference to me. You know how in the kitchen, right next to the sink, you usually have a drawer for utensils with a cabinet above? Well, I had them removed, and I clearly remember the woman who sold us the condo saying, "Are you crazy?" People don't understand that when you walk with a walker, it's hell trying to carry your food to the table. I needed that drawer space out of my way so I could have easy access to a barstool right there to eat my meals. My helpful barstool is a feasible distance from the fridge and other nearby drawers. In fact, most nights ten years later, I still eat on my barstool. So do you think I'm crazy?

All this stuff for the last several pages happened around the age of, yup, you guessed it, twenty-five. Some of these incidents occurred slightly before, some slightly after. Life is always full for me.

I moved into my townhouse on July 26, 1998, and I started graduate school in September of that year. By the way, July 26 is the anniversary of *The American with Disabilities Act,* which had been passed in 1990. Cosmic coincidence.

My parents were bursting with pride that I had graduated from Ramapo with honors. As a college student, I had had extended time on tests, and a scribe for notes and papers. I share this because although I have an academically strong photographic mind, I still need these accommodations, not unlike accommodations for someone who is blind or Deaf or has paraplegia or any disability. My busy mind combined with these accommodations helped me to earn a grade point average of 3.7 upon graduation. My glowing mother and father thought that was the final destination concerning my big accomplishments in life. Little did they know that in a few years I would obtain a Master's degree in Counseling, again with high honors. I guess I was suited for higher learning after all, despite what I had been told once upon by that lady at Rider University.

The generous gifts that I received from friends and relatives for my graduation from Ramapo were like shower gifts for my condo. That's why, years later, when I got married, I didn't want a bridal shower. In addition to my own domestic stuff, Mac had his piles of domestic stuff, too. I hate bridal showers and baby showers so it was fine with me that Mac and I just didn't need any more stuff!

Concerning my area of study for my Master's, while relaxing one evening in my cozy condo-townhouse, I clearly recall reading a book about psychotherapy that intrigued me. It was galvanizing. It was everything I had missed as an undergrad. The techniques, the analytical series, and the terminology blew my mind! It was right then and there that I decided to pursue my Master's degree from Seton Hall in Counseling. And it turned out that in grad school it was somewhat easier than being an undergrad because there were no tests, just papers galore. Okay, it wasn't that easy. Back then, research was just beginning—I mean, really just beginning--to be accessed by the masses via the Internet. Nevertheless, most of my research was obtained the old-fashioned way.

I've already explained this technique to you. Needless to say, I just can't understand why my students wimp out and complain about research nowadays. They have the Internet at their fingertips!

The first professor I had at Seton Hall, Dr. Dolores Thompson, was a terrific teacher and mentor. Unfortunately, she left after my first year, which saddened me because she was the one who had first urged me to apply to the counseling program.

That initial year of grad school was enormously challenging. The classes were extraordinarily rigorous, and the amount of work was unbelievable; however, I really wanted to become a psychotherapist. When Dr. Thompson left, Dr. H became my new advisor. I must say, he was a very attractive advisor. Regrettably, despite being dashingly handsome, he didn't know what the hell he was doing. To get me out of his hair and to do something positive for my education, he placed me in an internship at the a inner city school

As a result, I continued my studies at Seton Hall University while acting as a counselor at this school for young people with all kinds of disabilities, ages three to twenty-one. Although the legislation was in place for these students with disabilities to attend "regular" school, society was (and remains) in transitional desegregation.

The school exclusively for students with disabilities, and with, fortunately, a wide spectrum of ethnicities represented. These kids were wonderful, but the staff was mostly horrible. With few exceptions, I experienced a regression in attitude in regard to working with me, a professional with a disability. All of the teachers and administrators were non-disabled. I was told that I could not eat in the cafeteria (my poor coordination and resultant "messy" eating disturbed some people), so I ate in a room by myself. This was post-ADA and completely illegal, but I was told that if I did not like it, I could leave. I loved my students and wanted to stay, so I did not buck the system. I did, however, switch supervisors the next year, and she "allowed" me to eat in the cafeteria.

At Seton Hall, I remained diligent, but I had a difficult time with my advisors. They had never had a Master's degree candidate who had a major disability. Again, due to the fact that I really loved the kids at the school, I stayed the course at Seton Hall. One of the problems was that one of my non-disabled advisors from Seton Hall knew of my troubles at the school for students with disabilities, and out of concern for me, she advised me to leave the School. I explained that these students had never had a professional adult role model with a major disability, and, therefore, it was imperative that I stay. This was hard for my non-disabled advisor to comprehend, but we eventually agreed to my staying at the School for two years. It was difficult--and spectacularly worthwhile.

Just to enlighten you as to the prejudices at the school, my on-site supervisor, a non-disabled man, said to me that he truly loved helping the crippled children. I said, "Excuse me?" I knew what he meant because he lived it. He was condescending and paternalistic to the young people, getting his own feel-good jollies and not working to empower his students. Yes, indeed, attitudes are the biggest disabilities.

As for the other staff at they treated the kids unprofessionally. Trust me, it was a horrible staff with the exception of a handful of people. My daily thirty-five minute drive actually took me forty to fifty years back in time. These "professionals" did not understand the Disability Rights Movement at all. And here I come, an energetic young woman with only my personal experiences and my academic credentials in hand. Right-minded as I was, even I lacked intimate connection with children with disabilities. That soon changed.

A typical day was a stressful one. The second year I was there, I begged and pleaded to get my own office. They gave me an office, all right--the closet next to the sink! Depending on the age of the reader, you will know what kind of desk I had. It was one from the 1950s, little more than a broken-ass chair. It was cream-colored, with a little space to put your books below the table. I had no filing cabinet. And a student who was ambulatory had to sit on a little step just to talk to me. Students in wheelchairs fortunately *had* their own chairs. Weren't they lucky? Disability sometimes has its benefits.

Today as I speed down the hall on my electric scooter from my own *real* office to my appointment with Mike Fluhr, he calls out to me, "I got your coffee, but I forgot your straw!"

Man, life is a dream. That straw should be my biggest problem.

I shout back, "They're in 'my' drawer!" Even though I have my own office, I still have a drawer in Mike's office. The comfortable office arrangement I have today at Ramapo is the polar opposite of my pitiful office. Man, I climbed the staircase of oppression every day at that school. Writing this memoir reminds me of all the rotten places I've been. That staircase never leaves my mind.

Let me escort you into my typical day. To maintain confidentiality, I refer to my students by alphabet letters.

As I open my appointment book, which Dr. Chang had given me, I am thinking to myself, "I hate Thursdays." I have four kids who are coming for individual counseling sessions, and I run an adolescent group in the afternoon. The topic is Sex Education, because many of the students engage in inappropriate sexual behavior. I'll tell you about some of the kids I worked with. Right on time, W enters my office without even a knock! I say, "Go back out, close that damn door, and give it a knock; otherwise you're not coming in."

"Why do you gotta be a pain in the ass, Miss K?"

"Because I'm here to teach you something for the real world. Knocking is one of them." He knocks, then re-enters.

"Can I sit on your scooter? This step is uncomfortable."

"Sorry, no."

W is an unusual adolescent kid with a disability. Ed Roberts, who is famous as the Father of the Independent Living Movement, believed that kids with disabilities lacked street smarts due to their overprotected lives. W was the exception. He had been molested by his biological father, and, in turn, W had molested his sister. He was at home in "the hood." My counseling techniques with him were not the patronizing techniques that other counselors used. My methodology was right on his level. The only one who used similar dynamics was the six-foot-six African American social worker on our counseling team. I was in good company there.

I had a total of fourteen sessions with W. He said to me, "You really understand—like no one else." I eventually fought to take him in as a foster child. For that to happen, there was an initial investigation into W's home life. The investigation by the social worker revealed that his current foster parents were abusing him. Unfortunately, this is not unusual for foster parents of disabled kids. I lost the case, and it broke my heart. Nevertheless, in our counseling sessions, I remained tough on him. I was reprimanded by the School Coordinator and told, "You really don't know how to handle disabled inner-city kids without cognitive problems." What? Oh God, save me from this all-knowing, benevolent-adult idiocy.

Okay, back to the other kids I counseled. I had fifteen minutes for each "client," that allocated time being expressly devised for my SOAP report. You're probably saying, "SOAP? What's that?" *Subjective/ Objective/Action Plan;* my snapshot viewpoint. I was to devise both a purely clinical viewpoint and an overall lesson plan for each student. Sounds great, but as I said, I only had fifteen minutes a day with any given kid. By the time we had broken the ice, it was time for them to leave. Very demoralizing for them and for me.

Tap tap. I heard a soft knock at my door.

"Come in, C. Here take my chair. I'll sit on the step." "C" had been one of my first clients, and one of the great teachers in my life. C had been absolutely, completely mute for five years, and she was acting out in class. I had been seeing her since my first year, and we continued into my second year. Patience was the key. She wouldn't talk to me for three sessions. She just colored. I asked her very few questions during these sessions, but I provided her with a calm, safe haven with a disabled mentor who cared. During the fourth session, she drew a picture of her family. "Miss K, that's my mommy. That's my daddy—who hits me. And that's my brother. I gotta go now." Wow. My jaw dropped. I had hoped C would start talking, but it was still overwhelming to witness.

Every Tuesday, I had a meeting with my first direct superior, Lee. When I recounted to him the speaking incident with C, we concurred that this was a *major* breakthrough in my counseling career. The problem was that C only wanted to talk with me. I told Dr. Lee I hadn't done anything wonderful; I had just sat there patiently. Pure, undemanding peace and quiet. Apparently that's what she needed. C told me everything, and at the end she was beginning to talk with her classmates.

One time she said, without emotion, "I don't talk because I don't like my body."

I thought to myself, "Good Lord, there must be so many women with disabilities who feel the same way. Women and girls who feel as if they're in competition with the 'perfect' able-bodied women." Of course I understand that non-disabled women also suffer from poor body image due to the media's "perfect" role models. Nevertheless, I believe it is often more difficult for women with disabilities. I scribbled my thoughts on the beauty of the disabled form and proceeded to talk with C about it. When she left my office, I knew continuing to address this issue was of the utmost importance.

As I was writing my closing notes about C, my third client knocked energetically on the door.

"I'm so happy to see you, Miss K! I have a crush on a boy. His name is E! I tried to hold his hand, and I kissed him. But he ran away. He's so cute."

I experienced a lot of countertransference with students at this school. This client was exactly like I had been as a teenager. However, I now knew appropriate sexual behavior, whereas she did not, just like many sixteen-year-olds. When she spoke, I heard the subtext, "He isn't interested in me, and I don't know why." I knew this boy had a girlfriend already, so we talked about that, and more.

Ed Roberts said that it is quite common for many adolescents with disabilities to be uneducated about sex. The outgrowth is often inappropriate behavior as hormonal teenagers and, later, as adults.

I was left all alone in my mini-sessions to deal with this monumental issue. I spoke from the heart and did my best. It was a bumpy ride, but I do know that my clients liked the honesty of the friendly, safe place I provided.

While all this stuff was going on at, I was still taking classes on the Seton Hall campus. As usual, I had an able-bodied schedule and a disabled body--more very tough stairs to climb as I once again experienced the difficulties of keeping up with the able-bodied world. Many people consider me intelligent and my problems have never been keeping up with coursework. But in this instance, the problem *was* maintaining my physical and emotional health to finally earn my Master's.

Positive aspects about Seton Hall included the fact that I was academically challenged. Gone were the days when I was bored in classes. The demands were high, and I met the challenges. My professors and advisors did not consider my disability to be the primary issue, but instead, the emphasis was on my education. This time around in grad school, necessary accommodations like extra time on tests and a scribe was not needed because the work was done on my own time at my own pace. Again, I graduated with high honors. My tenacity paid off.

At the same time I was succeeding in my program, I was dealing with something crucial on a regular basis. I haven't told you about the panic attacks and clinical depression I've had ever since I was a little kid. When the damn panic attacks consume me, I feel raw, shitty, frail, and frightened. Add clinical depression to that and at such times, I'm beyond miserable. Enough said. You might wonder, "How the hell do you cope?" Well, I just weather the panic attacks. I actually compartmentalize them and kinda forget them. I guess that's called denial. It's also called survival. I'm compelled to remember full force when the next panic attack happens, just when I least expect it. That stinks.

So, what are the secrets to my success? Trying to be humble and living a modest life are two "secrets." I have a good, healthy sense of humor. And I don't let anyone or anything stop me. During the quest for my Master's, the fascinating course of study propelled me forward.

My personal life propelled me forward, as well. I met up with Ken the drummer again. Old feelings never go away, at least not for me. Honestly, we did not "hook up." It was the true closure that I needed; however, several years later, I actually bumped into him again. Ken and I are very similar in a lot of ways. We both have CP. We're both ambitious. We're both too smart for own good, and we *like* to get in trouble. But most of all, we both want to help the disabled community—each in our unique way: me as a scholar and Ken as an artist.

As I'm preparing for my class this particular afternoon at Ramapo, I hear two familiar voices. Oh, shit, Mike S. --and that just can't be Ken! They don't even knock on my door; they just barge in like fifteen years ago (but back then, it was my dorm room). Ken says, "Damn, you're a geek now, but you're moving up in the world!" He spots my Bob Marley hat hanging in the office.

Mike S., an old buddy of ours from back in the day, declares, "It took her six years to get a freakin' office. Leave that woman alone."

"Man, you've got books like a geek," Ken retorted.

We talk for five or ten minutes, and then back to work I go with my typist.

During my time at Seton Hall, I fired my first live-in housekeeper, whom I will call O. She was a lazy bum. Living in my townhouse did not present a lot of work to do. Honestly, you could be done in two hours and get a second job, too. Not so for this housekeeper. She just plopped down and stayed there. You might wonder why I kept her so long. I have to admit, I kept waiting for her to clean up her act—excuse the pun. I believe in second, even third chances. I've been given second and third chances, which helped me move from being a raucous, teenage college student to a respectable woman with a Master's degree.

I knew O because she had been my PCA during my last year at Ramapo. She wanted to get out of her parents' place, and I needed someone to help me out. But she was so damn lazy that she was in her room watching TV most of the day. That just didn't sit well with me. We both knew it wasn't a good situation, and we managed to end on a friendly note. She was a genuinely good soul with lazy habits.

While I was at Seton Hall, I had the good fortune to fly off to Jamaica with my whole family. It was a well-deserved rest. My parents rented a beautiful villa with a private chef and butler. It was like a fantastic dream. I surprised myself that first night and ate my dinner like a meek Daddy's little girl. I remember asking my father's permission to leave the table, just as if I were a child. I was not feeling well. I fell asleep at six o' clock and woke up the next morning coughing. It was dreadful. I called out for my brother Charlie to help me, but he couldn't do much. They rushed me to the hospital and found out that I had developed bronchitis—a recurring and painful illness in my life. It was horrendous. I was in this beautiful house with a beautiful pool, a beautiful beach, a butler, a cook, and a maid, and I was in my damn bed watching every Jamaican TV show there was. My best friend became the butler. Tea and honey never tasted so good. My family remarked that I looked like hell, and they weren't lying. I needed Mac there at that time to help me cough up the mucous, but we hadn't yet met.

I'm sitting here today with bronchitis, having just returned from Mexico with Mac and I feel like shit all over again, despite the fact that Mac *has* helped me cough up mucous. I have always hated to be sick.

While we were in Jamaica, nobody in my family could understand why I wanted to finish my Master's. I felt like I was seventeen again, being informed that it was impossible to obtain my driver's license. After all my hard work at higher education, I saw the staircase of oppression looming before me yet again, this time put in the picture by the loving but misguided concerns of my family. I knew it would be difficult to keep climbing, but the end would be worth it.

I knew I couldn't teach a college-level course without a Master's, and I wanted to teach on the college level with all my heart. So I remained vigilant, in spite of my family's words to me about taking it easy. Sometimes I just know I'm absolutely, completely right, and this was one of those times. How did I see the big picture in spite of the enormous pressure? It's at such times I almost hear myself: "Only you, Christine."

I don't have very high self-esteem, despite my accomplishments. My low self-esteem is a constant factor in my life. But I'm a great professor and I'm great at my job, and I know I have that to offer the world. That's where my self-esteem positively shines.

When my intern hours at A. Harry Moore were over, I finally had a little time to breathe. And I do mean literally to breathe. Hallelujah! My bronchitis cleared up, momentarily. There were no summer classes that I needed to take. I was stress free and, of course, up to trouble.

Wanna know what I was doing? Okay, just relax and listen up. It's a little steamy, as usual.

Well, it didn't start out steamy. I was dating this man named David. He was so sweet--and so immature. He didn't drive. He had CP. And it was nice just to communicate with him. We only kissed. He met my parents, and my family adored him. Wise old friend Sandy hated him, but he *was* sweet. It's just that there was no fire between us. I held onto the relationship solely to occupy my time.

I was also hanging out with a guy named Pete. It was the strangest relationship I've ever had. We went out to eat at least three times a week. We acted like a couple. You'd think we were married! I swear I gave him so many chances to kiss me, but he never did. We never even held each other, but we flirted like hell. My mom and sister were crazy about him. He even played golf with them, which was a big deal. But he never kissed me. Nothing. Was he gay? Was that the man I was supposed to marry? I don't know. He was one strange dude, and, ironically, we clicked. Remember, I like offbeat. Unusual works for me. And true to the quirkiness of our flirty but platonic relationship, for Christmas he gave me books about true love.

You know, I sometimes think Mac is gonna file for divorce after he reads this book. (Just kidding. Mac has his past, too, and what matters most is *now*—the two of us living happily in the present.) Nevertheless, men, men, men—too many men. But according to my standards, I wasn't actually dating Pete because we had no physical contact. Like I said, it was strange.

David and I had a big fight. We were on again and off again.

Meanwhile, my now-longtime colleague Ms. Wexler had come down to my condo for the weekend. We had a wonderful time talking about everything, including the fact that I had a year left of graduate school. She suggested, "Why don't you co-teach First Year Seminar with me?" My good pal, the infamous Dr. Patrick Chang was in charge of the program! But by now I had a great relationship with him, which had eclipsed my undergraduate follies. Still, that meant I would be teaching *and* going to grad school.

"Okay, but only one semester."

Guess what? This is my sixth year, and I now have my own office. Looking back, it was a laborious journey to get where I am today. It might not last long, but I'm here now. When they kick me out, I'll take photos of my office as proof of my presence!

Yes, one semester teaching First Year Seminar ended up being six years. And I hope it'll be twenty more years. I was so excited to teach, but I didn't realize how demanding it was. Miss Wexler was the lead instructor, so the workload was not as taxing as it is now. During these six years of teaching, my life has been hectic, confusing, and just plain crazy. But it's just as often completely wonderful and rewarding in my roles as devoted teacher and wife.

The Stairway to Adulthood

Ever wonder if you could take a day back and re-live it differently? Would you? Let me tell you something. The nineteenth of August in 2001 is the one day I would take back and do all over again. I remember that fateful day so clearly. It was insane. The night before, I had gone to my cousin's for a party and drove home drunk. Not good, I know. Ironically I got home safe and sound. However, the next day a tempest started that I've always wished I could have avoided. That day was the day I was introduced to my "drug of choice." At the onset, I was twenty-seven years old, and my addicted misery continued up to the age of thirty, when I was suddenly, mercifully saved from myself.

Many people think addiction is related only to drugs and alcohol. Naturally, that's the first thing that comes to mind, but there are plenty of addictions out there, believe me. Remember, I'm a licensed therapist, and I know these things. My addiction was Nick Rick.

The phone rang, waking me from sleep. My head was throbbing and I was quite annoyed. It was my mom, saying that someone wanted to talk to me. A voice got on the line. I said, "Ken? Is that you? How the hell did you get to my parents' house?"

"Who the hell is Ken?"

"Then who are you?"

"Take a wild guess."

I did. It was "Nick Rick," one of my childhood buddies. I was still in my pj's as he announced, "I'm on my way to see you." My parents proceeded to give him directions to my house.

I remember exactly what I was wearing and where I was sitting when Nick Rick approached the door. Some people believe in love at first sight. I swear it was love/addiction at first sight. He came in, and we talked for hours. I think five hours to be exact. I was leaving for Las Vegas for a fiftieth birthday celebration the next day. It was for Lorraine, my mom's good friend. He said, "Call me tonight." I wasn't gonna call his ass. No way.

When I got back, there was a message from him. We talked on the phone for hours. The next day he came over, and the passion that ensued was unbelievable! After that, he was off to Fairleigh Dickinson University in Teaneck. He had two years left to finish his bachelor's degree. Every Friday night, he would swing by and spend the weekend with me. It was kinda weird because for all the times he came to my townhouse, I rarely went to his campus, or even out to dinner with him. If I had a man-making machine, I would put Pete and Nick Rick into it to create the perfect mate. The sex was good with Nick Rick, and I went out and had a good time with Pete. Damn. But of course, there is no such machine. Well, at least there wasn't then. Today I am blessed with Mac. Believe me, I mean blessed.

Nick Rick and I never left the house. We continued to our thing. The oddest thing is that I really felt loved by him. He made me feel so "on top of the world." But he never wanted to visit my parents or be officially introduced to the rest of my family. Likewise, I didn't care to have anything to do with his family. I remember teaching at Ramapo and later visiting him on his campus. We were in his car later that day and he told me that he didn't like to kiss. Here I was on his campus, and he didn't even take me into his dorm! I told this to Sandy, and she replied, "He's a player."

I thought, "I feel love from him." But, in November, I started to feel like a whore. I started to give him money, whenever he asked for it. I can't even tell you how much. I bought him a PlayStation for Christmas, which was a big deal. Then he broke up with me because he didn't want to spend New Year's Eve with me. Next, in a complete reversal, he called me on New Year's Eve to hang out with me. At my place, as usual. Episodes like this went on and on. My love/addiction grew deeper and deeper.

When I graduated from Seton Hall, he didn't bother to come to my graduation.

Oh, and I still I haven't been to his dorm room.

We moved on to a weirder pattern. He came to my home on Friday nights at two in the morning. Then at six in the morning, he vanished. But I still thought that he was in love with me, because I was feeling that addictive high. It was exhilarating and fantastic and I chased it for years. Eventually, that elusive high morphed into depression.

For the record, I was twenty-seven years old. Emotionally, I stayed that age for the next several years. My life seemed to prosper, but psychologically, I was mired. It was not booze or drugs because their allure had pretty much dissipated, (Not so for him.) My horrific addiction was my unhealthy relationship. It lasted two years.

That addiction/love got stronger and stronger when we were together—that is, physically together, even though we had no formal relationship. He always asked me for a lot of money, and I handed it over to him. That situation got worse. His temper was out of control. He was drunk all the time, and I was not. But I felt the love, or did I feel the high? I was controlling because I always wanted to know where he was and what he was doing. In turn, he was verbally and sexually abusive. What I had left of my bruised self-esteem disappeared completely. This was all going on while I was finishing up grad school.

To this day, I'm trying to figure out if our relationship was an addiction or true love. I haven't felt that connection with another soul in my life. I continue to struggle with that issue, and at times it seems like unbelievable fiction. I know it wasn't.

You know why we got "divorced"? (In my mind, we were married.) I had purchased a BMW-X5 for him, and he sent me a little bouquet of flowers. It was January. The next month, on Valentine's Day, he didn't even give me a card or anything else. I rode in that BMW a total of three times! My parents found out about everything, and that was the day I tried to commit suicide. April 16, 2003. I was very sick and depressed, psychologically and emotionally. I felt useless and that I had nothing to live for. In my twisted thinking, I was doing the world a favor by doing away with myself.

Not long after Mom had happily re-introduced me to Nick Rick, my parents saw through him. In due time, they did not like Nick Rick, but they put up with us. I'm not saying that we all sat down and broke bread together. No way. In a moment of clarity, my dad proclaimed sarcastically, "I hope you get married to Nick Rick someday." Why? Because Dad knew I "loved him" but he knew Nick Rick would never marry me. Dad saw right through him.

An actively addicted person cannot see reality. However, I fleetingly glimpsed it when he did not celebrate our second anniversary and later, when he wanted to break up with me. Next, he demanded that I pay his car insurance.

"Hell, no! I've only been in that freakin' car three times! You want *me* to pay *your* car insurance? It's my car, anyway!"

I am currently in therapy, and that is why. My therapist helps me so much to gain some insight to this addiction, as she plainly calls it.

Mom says, "You married the perfect man. Who else would put up with your demanding bullshit?"

Mom is right. I did marry the perfect man.

As expected, my cell phone rings right now, precisely fifteen minutes before class. Mac is on the line. "I got reservations for 9:30 tonight at the Thai place."

"Okay, I gotta run to class. Love you."

"Love you more."

I get up from my desk, gather my books, say good-bye to the typist, and off I go to teach. Identity Formation is topic of the day, but you remember that from our discussion at home when Mac was yodeling about the resplendent day.

On the way to the classroom, I mull over the fact that my parents truly adore Mac. He's hardworking. He pays the bills. We do things together. He never asks me for money, even though I have my trust fund. We eat breakfast together every single day because with our hectic schedules that's the one time we can sit together peacefully, talking and enjoying each other's company. My siblings say the exact same thing as our parents, that he's wonderful. And he is.

Dammit, that doesn't stop me from being an addict, even though I'm currently in a healthy remission, one that I hope will last forever, each day at a time. Sometimes I get thoroughly confused and upset about the whole mess.

I'm sure you've surmised how I'm feeling today. It's a lovely autumn day outside, but I feel depressed. The trees are in spectacular display, and I feel empty. My zest for life is dormant this afternoon.

My view of love is that it is a paradox. I think I'm due for my period tomorrow. I'm sad, but so much around me is good—actually fantastic beyond my wildest dreams. In fact, a true miracle has occurred. My brother's brain tumor is gone after only three months of chemotherapy. He still has to go into isolation for three weeks for something to do with stem cells.

Two days ago, I must tell you, this is a dream come true. I haven't yet started the long process of creating the curriculum, but just having it approved (and having my own office) is bliss to me. Despite my cursing and whining, I really am an academic at heart. Scoring this *coup* is the result of years of academic work. I am so proud.

Why am I sad today? Plain and simple--PMS is a bitch.

As I said, I'm seeing a terrific therapist. What makes her so wonderful is that she is unlike all the therapists I have seen in the past, who viewed me as a Super Crip, totally disregarding my freaked-up feelings and huge pile of emotional baggage. All those therapists simply concentrated on how "amazing" I was, and how they were so "impressed" by me. Many people laud me with, "You're so inspirational!" I hate that. I have accomplished a great deal, but I'm still a wee bit nuts. (I want to address that with my therapist!) If I wanted to hear a slightly different version of how inspirational I am, I'd just go to my office and meet with my students. Although they think I'm terrific, they must also think I'm naive. When they do poorly in my class, they think if they give me compliments, they'll get an "A." Wrong! So I don't need the compliments from a therapist either, I need to understand my issues!

My current therapist calls me a spoiled brat and says that Nick Rick was most assuredly an addiction. She has helped me to realize that with all my successes, I still feel the need to debase myself. That deplorable mentality or behavior is not at all uncommon. Just think of New York governor Eliot Spitzer, Senator Larry Craig, 1920s religious leader Aimee Semple McPherson, or anyone who has fallen from their pedestal in disgrace. The ecstasy and agony. My therapist is extraordinarily helpful. We work steadfastly to help me live free of active addiction.

Back then, during the years I spent with Nick Rick, it seemed as if my whole life revolved around him. It did to some extent, but, mercifully, other things happened, as well.

In my family, it seems to happen that whenever a person dies, literally or figuratively, another person is brought into the world. During the psycho-honeymoon stage of Nick Rick, my sweet niece Nina was born. Everyone was deliriously happy. At the same time, my grandfather was dying. I would visit him in the hospital every day after Seton Hall. I read my boring statistics book to him while he was sleeping. When he awoke, he would say, "Read me some of that shit." I know my grandfather and I had a very strong bond because as I write this I am experiencing a unique tingling sensation. So far, it's only Grandpa with whom I have had that supernatural connection. Like me, my grandfather was a real pistol. In the hospital, he called my dad and told him, "Get me out of this hospital so I can go to the bar one last time." And that's just what Dad did.

Not much later, on a Tuesday morning in October, my mom came over to my house to do my laundry. I said to her, "Meet me at the hospital at four, and bring Grandma, too." The previous night, my grandfather had said to me, "You are my pride and joy. Remember when you drove me to Sears way back when? I was so proud of you, and I always will be. Don't tell anyone that I know my time is near. I just need to see my wife, my oldest daughter, and you tomorrow." I honored his request to bring the people he most wanted to see. Mom, my grandma, and I got to say our heartfelt good-byes. He whispered, "Thank you."

The following morning at six o'clock, I got a call from my mom. I said, "I know, and I'm sorry, too."

The funeral was awful. When I die, I never want to be stuck in a freakin' coffin because it costs too much. My last image of my grandfather was of him in that wretched coffin with ungodly make-up on his face. My mom was kneeling next to the coffin, as I was, and we were crying hysterically. I've informed my family that when I die, I want the cheapest funeral possible, because I believe in reincarnation. I think a roaring party in celebration of all the good in my life would be more in order! I cried so much at Grandpa's funeral, and that's when I first started to feel the tingling sensation. Then, as now, I believe it to be my grandfather's soul. To me, that means he's not reincarnated yet. I know he'll never leave me because I'll recreate him in my mind for the duration of my life on this planet.

People say they have funerals for closure. Well, my final wishes are that I want people to come to my house and have an extra strong drink and yap about whatever they want. I don't want anyone crying for me. If someone does cry, my soul will be announcing, "And you fools are crying? Don't! I'm in a better place."

During the grieving stage for my grandfather, which lasted six months, Nick Rick wanted me to get over it fast so he can come over.

On an educational level, life got easier, which afforded me the temporary luxury of finishing my Master's program. Nick Rick and I were doing "fine." (You know, Freaked up-Insecure-Neurotic-Emotional.) In fact, everything was relatively easygoing. At that time, I was finishing my thesis on countertransference in order to become a licensed therapist (uniquely, a licensed therapist with a disability). I was required to write thirty-five pages with fifteen citations. Okay, I could do that, no problem. However, there were two weeks in May I'll never forget. My plans were to attain my degree at the end of the summer, so I had to take two classes that spring. One was entitled "Group Therapy." Boy oh boy, that class trained me very well in how to run a group therapy session. The class met five times a week, for four hours each. I was expecting to simply walk into the Group Therapy classroom with a syllabus handed to me. I was expecting the professor to start the lecture, as usual. This was not the case, at all. Dr. Smith just sat there with twelve of us doctoral students looking at each other. We were quiet and well behaved. One of my peers inquired politely after fifteen minutes, "Well, are we gonna start class?"

The professor replied, "We have started class." That class turned out to be the most intense two weeks in my life. He ran the class as a group therapy session. Then we went home and wrote about the techniques that were utilized in each session. It was the most amazing, enlightening experience. The first day, we were polite toward one another, but as the days went by, hostility between us grew. It was group therapy at its best. By the end of two weeks, we simultaneously hated each other and were good friends. This was because we all knew each other's shit. We kept

111

in touch for a while, but then those relationships faded away. That was my best class and the last class I had to complete.

I'd finished all my work and received my Master's degree. My parents were so happy, and so was I. Naturally, I was joyful getting that diploma. I had worked so damn hard for my Master's but when I read it I was shocked to see it was in Latin. All that work, and I couldn't even read the damn thing.

As a gift, my parents rented me a condo on the beach at the Jersey shore for five weeks. I thought that it would be awesome. Nick Rick and I could be together for at least three weeks. My family could come down, too—just not at the same time as Nick Rick. The condo was on the Point Pleasant boardwalk. We could easily go to the tiki bar and get drunk. Of course, that scenario never happened. Nick Rick came down for four nights, that's it. We had a helluva time, and he still says that was the greatest time of his life. My sister came down every weekend. Aunt Kathy and her daughter came down, as well. But I soon learned something. Having a house down at the shore was more aggravation than it was worth. It seemed that, after a short time, nobody came to visit me. I sometimes secretly drove home to my townhouse.

One night, I was so bored that I went to the club on the boardwalk by myself, and I twisted my damn ankle.

On a brighter note, my Aunt Gina lived by the boardwalk; I went to her house for dinner at least three times a week. She noticed that my ankle was badly sprained and took me to the hospital. My parents were away somewhere. My sister kindly packed up everything from the shore house and took it to my condo. It was the end of the summer.

I was going to teach my first course, solo. I taught First Year Seminar, and the topic was "Values." I had no clue what I was doing. However, the kids were sweet, and I enjoyed teaching. The paradoxes in my life—the addiction of Nick Rick and the joy of teaching in a professional capacity—were strangely intriguing to me.

Have you ever awakened in the morning and thought it was just going to be another boring day? For me, "boring" meant simply going to work, teaching a class, and coming home, just a regular day. Well, the day I'm going to share with you right now wasn't a regular day at all. It was one of the most notable days on the staircase of my career life. As usual, I was pissed off at Nick Rick and almost ran over . Mike

Fluhr on campus. Covering my pissed-off attitude, I chirped perkily, "Hi! Don't I know you from somewhere?"

"Yes, you were a Peer when I was teaching College Seminar. How are you?"

Blah, blah, blah.

He informed me that he was teaching "Self Growth."

"Can I be your Peer?" I figured the extra work was for only one day a week, and I could do counseling on the side.

As it turned out, after teaching two classes that semester, I found I liked the academic atmosphere and I never went back to counseling. I knew I wasn't going to get paid at first for my teaching, but I wanted to get through the academic door at Ramapo. Maybe I would, and maybe I wouldn't get paid to do this someday. But sometimes you have to take a chance.

As for teaching with Mike, it was a fantastic learning experience for me, and it was arduous, as well. I worked my ass off for him. I remember that one time after class we were sitting in the Pay Caf having coffee when he asked me, "If you could teach one class, what would it be?"

While co-teaching for a semester, we had built up a good rapport.

"Bullshit. I want to teach a course about the bullshit in the world, and how to navigate the bullshit," was my smart-ass reply.

"Really? Come on now,

I said, "Okay, on a serious note. There's a great, cutting-edge discipline called Disability Studies. My dream is to teach a course on Disability Studies." And so began the first of many conversations I had with him on this course I wanted to develop.

"Well, kiddo, you do the research, and I'll support it if it's good-- but I know it'll be good because you are a pretty good professor. Okay, really good."

"Are you shittin' me?"

"Actually, no."

I went home and did all my research. I knew there was a Society for Disability Studies, and I soon joined. I learned that a conference was planned for the middle of June, and it was now May of 2003. I asked my mom, as usual, if she would come with me. No, let me correct that. I said to my mom, "I'm driving by myself to the conference in Maryland."

"The hell you are. I'm coming with you." Mom had every right to be concerned. This was only one month after my suicide attempt.

My mom, I have never known another woman like her, who has completely dedicated her life to her four children. Yes, we are opposites, but I admire her dedication in literally giving up her life for her children. To this very day, that has never changed. Nor does she think she gave up her life. She's a totally awesome, hard-working mom.

I answered her comment about coming with me, "Mom, you're the most dedicated, loving, and sometimes overbearing mother that anyone is lucky to have." If I didn't say "overbearing," it would have been a Hallmark story, but this is no Hallmark story.

This evening I roll into my classroom as "Professor Dearest." I hate coming into a classroom and starting right in on a lecture. Other professors that I know, like Mike, just take attendance at the beginning, and then start in right away. My style is unique. I ask everyone, "How are you doing?" Then, I crack a few stupid jokes. While I go through my jokes, I bring up my Power Point. I really hate it when professors give detailed email notes to their students, because then the students get bored in the class. Although I email some material to my students, the Power Points serve as a guide for them to keep on track, given my speech impediment. I pose questions in between lectures, that way I can see if they actually understand me. I continue to make stupid-ass jokes, which also serve as feedback for me. If only two or three students are laughing, then I ask them what I just said. I make sure everyone understands my CP accent. It is my responsibility to deliver the information the best I can. However, as college students, they must realize that this is part of their education, as well. I try to create a comfortable atmosphere with all my classes and not intimidate anyone, unlike some professors who keep their distance. It's a bit strenuous trying to please all my students, but I honestly do my best.

I challenge you to go to ratemyprofessor.com. I get excellent reviews and I get terrible reviews. And then, I cry. How can you be a good professor? The reviews complain about how students get kicked out of my class because they are texting. This is a pet peeve of mine. It's disrespectful, and I hate it. So some students write bad reviews.

The good reviews say that I'm an excellent teacher, kind hearted and approachable. They also like that we interact with one another. I am thorough in my presentations. I get a natural high when I'm teaching. I feel that I'm on top of the staircase. But the staircase never ends. And then, the next day when I go to the mall, and people ask me, "Is your Mommy with you?" I regress a few steps. No, I regress more than a few steps. That kind of stuff leaves me emotionally empty.

My economic status is comfortable. I don't brag about the things I have. Actually, I'm the opposite. I don't shop for myself because I feel I don't need any more material things than what I have. Mac buys me clothes when I need new things. I'm serious in saying that I'm generally not a braggart—although Mac and my mom often say that I do brag about my job. A part of me can't believe that I have a wonderful career, with all the damn obstacles I've gone through. I'm finally up there. And yet, when I leave the office or the classroom or the campus, the oppression of the staircase is omnipresent.

Mom and I drove to Maryland to attend my first Disability Studies Conference. Most of the presentations went over my head; however, I still learned a lot. More important, I began to network with Mike Dorn from Temple University. He was a real mover and shaker in the field of Disability Studies.

I'll never forget how I met Mike, I mean the dignified Dr. Dorn. My mom unpacked while I went to the opening ceremony. The keynote speaker was Judy Heumann, a powerhouse in the Disability Movement. Afterward, I met Mom at the bar and informed her that I was stupid, because I didn't know what they were saying. She had had a couple of glasses of wine and replied, "You take after your mother. Want a glass of wine?"

There were two gentlemen next to us, who had attended the opening ceremony. I said to myself, "I might as well start networking now."

"Hi, my name is Christine Komoroski, and this is Mother Teresa."

They both laughed boisterously. In fact, they guffawed. At first, I couldn't figure out what was so outrageously funny. I had had four glasses of wine, and I soon realized they were buzzed, too. They were from Temple University and did, indeed, turn out to be a part of my Philadelphia networking.

As it turned out, I later trained at Temple University for a year. The first semester was excruciating. I drove two hours to Philadelphia to attend a post-grad class on Disability Culture on Thursday nights. Then, because I taught Freshman Seminar the next morning at Ramapo, I drove two hours home that night and the next morning I drove one hour from my house to Ramapo. Then I would teach my Freshman Seminar class and afterward, I drove home, another hour. I always crashed on those Fridays.

That November, Nick Rick and I had a huge argument. I had insomnia, which was worsening fast.

"I want to leave you. I was never in love with you." He was standing straight and tall in my foyer. He was expressionless.

In tears, crying hysterically, I screamed, "No! No!"

"We're not married. Get a grip."

From then on, things were never the same. Practically everything went downhill, although we still had our highs, just like a drug. He was both wastrel and, much more infrequently, a passionate lover.

He used to skip his Friday classes and surprise me on Thursday nights. We'd drink, and get high all weekend. After a time (I don't know how long), the mind-altering experiences with drugs and alcohol steadily decreased for me, while his steadily increased. But I didn't care because I knew the more stoned he got the longer he would stay with me. Or so I thought. We listened to Bob Marley most of the time, and we barbecued outside. He got bored, so he tried to fix up the basement. Yes, sometimes we were quite domestic. I genuinely thought that we would be married within a year, and soon thereafter, we'd have two kids: utopia at its best. But when he left on Sundays, it was horrible. I came off my high. Once a week, I experienced a major case of slipping and crashing down several steps, not even trying to pick myself up.

It was September 19, 2003, a day that I thought would be just another "normal" day. As usual, the stress of graduate school resulted in more respiratory problems for me. I was advised to see a pulmonologist after obtaining my Master's degree. The nightmare of my grad school schedule was over, and now I was going to see a doctor for my respiratory problem. Dr. Wolf advised me that there was a new vest on the market that helped to break up the mucus. The vest would come in the mail, and then a person would come and train me how to use it.

The phone rang. I didn't pick up because I was awash in tears. I knew the relationship with Nick Rick was disintegrating. For me, it was like an agonizing divorce. You know how couples have songs because it's romantic and lovey-dovey? Maybe that's not you, but that's what we had. When we broke up, I played all those songs and cried for days and days. That's how I handled the situation.

"Dammit to hell," I cursed, "that stupid-ass phone keeps ringing."

I got up from my bedroom and looked at the caller ID. Area code 808—I think that's Hawaii! Who the hell is in Hawaii? I bet it's his new girlfriend and he's in Hawaii with her, dammit.

"Let's hear about this drama," I said to myself. "Either he needs more money, or he's in jail; or he got killed, and it's an invitation to his funeral."

I actually relished the last choice. I listened to the voice on the machine. It was a calm, understated man with a sexy voice--he could talk to my machine all day!

"This is William McCohnell. They refer to me as Mac. I am the trainer for the vest company. Please call me back at your earliest convenience, and we can set up an appointment so I can train you on your vest. Dr. Wolf says you are very sick, and I need to come visit you as soon as possible. Thank you so much, and have a great day."

What, is this guy on pot? Sounds like a pothead—so calm, cool, and collected--and so sexy! I hated most men at this point so it was unusual for me to be attracted to a man's voice

"I'm not calling him back. I'll just get the damn vest and do it myself."

But that sexy voice kept calling me. Hmm, who was this man?

"Ms. Komoroski, I know you're very busy, but you're very sick, as well. I'm coming over Wednesday, September 19, at 1 o'clock. Please be there. My job is on the line. Just do this for me. It will take a half hour."

"Okay, okay! I guess I need to do this, for both of us," I thought to myself.

I called him right back.

"Dr. McCohnell, I'll be here, waiting for you, on the nineteenth."

"Thank you, Professor Komoroski."

(Who would have thought that three years later students would be calling me "Professor *McCohnell*"?)

On September nineteenth, the doorbell rang. I wasn't feeling well. No one was home, and I was letting a strange man into my house. What was I thinking? I let him in anyway. It was William McCohnell. He asked, "Where's the box?"

I said, "Right here."

He opened the box and said, "Do you have a VCR? You have to watch the tape with the vest on. The vest will make you cough up all the mucous and make you feel a lot better."

"Hell, no! I'm not doing that!"

He didn't know that Nick Rick used to scream and yell at me when I had to cough, so what could I do? Cough in front of a stranger? I explained to him why I wouldn't put the vest on. He explained to me that people cough in front of him every day, and that's his job. He "cured" them. He asked, "Do you have tissues?"

I asked myself, "Is this guy a miracle worker?"

Guess what--he *was* a miracle worker. After watching the tape he said, "I only need five more minutes of your time, and I'll be out." He informed me of a few more details about the vest and did the necessary paperwork.

I thought to myself, "This guy really is stupid. He's so calm that he's probably crazy. Thank God, he's leaving."

Little did I realize he was the wisest man I would ever know. He looked at my home and said, "Your house should be in a magazine."

A day later, I found out that I needed to have my wisdom teeth taken out. What? Oh no, no, no! I had a class to teach. There were too many things happening at once.

"We have to put you under to take your wisdom teeth out. You will have to stay overnight in the hospital due to the complications of CP," explained the nice oral surgeon.

I told Nick Rick I was scared. He promised, "Don't worry. I'll be there." Right. He never came. I had given this man a BMW, and he never even bothered to come to the hospital when I needed him. But of course who was there but my parents and Kim. Kim slept over that night. I was in so much pain that they gave me Percoset. I was crying to Kim that I was in horrific pain and that Nick Rick was on his way. I kept crying and crying. By the time the Percoset kicked in ten minutes later, she was feeding me chocolate pudding and I was high as a kite! Between sobs I proclaimed, "I like chocolate pudding! I like chocolate pudding!" And then I dozed off to sleep. Kim loves to tell that story.

I was mortified that Nick Rick hadn't bothered to take care of me, and he was driving around in that damn BMW.

As I got better that week, enjoying tons of chocolate pudding with Percoset, Nick Rick and I had the biggest fight. He wanted to break things off forever and ever this time. In disbelief, I pleaded, "Are you coming back?"

"Hell, no!"

"What about the car?"

He blasted, "Well, aren't you going to finish paying for it?" He had remained stubborn on that issue whenever I brought it up.

"You've got to be out of your freakin' mind! So you can drive the woman you're dating now, and she can make you feel good in my car? I don't think so, asshole. If you give me the payments and the insurance every month, then you can keep the goddam car. But I'm not paying for your car and your insurance just to be played a fool. "

I called my dad and told him the censored version of the story. "I told you I never liked him from the start. I told you he was a con artist. You have a lot of money, and he knows it. He doesn't love you, he loves your money. Can't you see that now?"

"Yes, Daddy, and I need your help. I need Mommy's help. Help me. Please help me." I was a five-year-old girl, lost in life. Would I ever wake up from this nightmare? I didn't know. I was at another five-year milestone, almost thirty years old, and I felt aged and completely defeated. My burning question was, "What should I do?"

I began with a little self-help. I, at long last, determined to break it off with Nick Rick. The enormity of the money issue had finally awakened me. I decided to stand my ground. I was actually proud of myself for that decision. Then I began to waver and inwardly bemoaned, "Only you, Christine. You got yourself into this mess. Now get yourself out of it."

"Everything's gonna be okay," I continued with my inner monologue. "I've got Mommy and Daddy to back me up—or maybe even get the car back for me." I knew my parents didn't like the fact that Nick Rick still had the car. I thought, "Maybe they'll intervene and bail me out because maybe they feel a little responsible." I know it sounds odd--and patronizing--on my part to revert to the guilt theory about parents of people with disabilities, but I assumed my parents would overprotect me on this issue. Guess what? They didn't. So I summoned my courage and determined to do my own dirty work. I wanted to break it off with Nick Rick emotionally and sexually. Looking back, I know those were good decisions, but they were exceedingly painful for me.

We all know that reality isn't linear. There are many events that meander through any given day or week or month. Such was the case with Nick Rick and my car. Almost before I knew it, weeks had passed, and I was back at school, teaching a class of fledgling eighteen-year-olds, who all wanted to talk with me after the first class. I sensed it was now or never with him. My students kept asking more and more questions. After chatting for about fifteen minutes, I politely excused myself and got out of there.

I zoomed home and met up with Nick Rick. I finally got the car, the keys, and my fragile sanity back. I said good-bye and good riddance.

Again, I am at Ramapo today. Again, my students are asking lots of questions. Usually, I stay around for quite awhile and chat with whomever wishes to further investigate the day's material, but today, I remind the class that their questions were answered on the syllabus, which had been emailed to them at the start of the semester. Quickly, I look at the clock on the wall. Tick, tick, tick.

"Shit, it's 8:30. I gotta get to the Thai restaurant in less than an hour!" I'm in such a hurry but thank God, I remember to take all my stuff with me like my pocketbook, keys, and my iPhone. I'm in my trusty van, and I'm off! I'm flying on 287, and my phone rings.

"Hello?"

It's Mac. "Take your time, honey. Don't speed. I'm leaving for the restaurant, and I'll be there soon. I'll just order your rack of lamb. Don't speed."

Ricky and Lucy are very competitive. I bet I can beat him there, even though he's at home, and the restaurant is only up the street for him. So, I put the pedal to the metal, and vroom down the highway, faster than usual, which is pretty damn fast.

Just a few years ago, speeding to Temple University was much more intense than beating Mac to the restaurant is now. Life is good, and my fast commute is fun, but at times I look back to 2003. I can't help doing so, I don't know why. I think about those gloomy events as I'm zooming along. On one such race, before I got the BMW back, I remember pulling off the highway and arguing on the phone with Nick Rick about the car. His famous line, whenever we were fighting about the future of "our baby," was always, "What am I? A freakin' fortuneteller? Get off my case."

"I guess not." Then I'd drive off, intimidated and in tears, to my class at Temple.

Why does this stuff still rent space in my head? It doesn't come up often, but it still does and it still has power to bother me.

Back to my recovery from getting my wisdom teeth removed.

I recall that when I returned home, I had received another message from that peaceful, sexy voice. "Ms. Komoroski, this is Mac. I need to come over because I lost the paperwork, and I need an original signature."

I said to myself, "Just what I thought. This guy is totally stupid." I called him back anyway and impatiently blurted, "Just fax it to me, and I'll fax it back."

"No, it will only take five minutes of your valuable time. And, as I said, I need an original signature."

He came over the following Monday. He was so nice, and he was cute. And he was so big. Light-skinned African American, and oh my God, have I mentioned that sexy voice? I asked him if he wanted a drink. He replied, "Okay. Water, please, no ice." We ended up talking for twenty minutes, during which time he informed me that he was going to Wyoming in three weeks. Since he was so nice, I asked him if he'd ever been to New York City. He replied, "No."

"I'll take you on a tour, if you want," I suggested. Yes, indeed, he was so kind that I had to make it up somehow for being so bitchy to him before.

"I'll get back to you," which he never did. I called him about our trip to the Big Apple, and he agreed to go with me. On October 18, 2003, I woke up thinking, "What in the world am I doing?"

I called Denise. "Should I go? I just broke up with Nick Rick!"

"You haven't been in a relationship for two years, you've been abused for two years. Go to New York City and have fun."

I was going to call and cancel with Mac, but he came a half hour early, so off we went to Manhattan.

Let me say that now, whenever we're in the van, he drives. Why? Because on that first date I drove fast and scared the hell out of him. I had never driven in New York City before, and I got so lost. The only parking garage I knew cost $60 an hour. "Okay, I'll pay it," I said to the garage attendant, but Mac refused to allow me to pay that much. I thought, "This guy is cheap. What's the big deal? I'm paying for the damn thing!" Just like the old TV show, *I Love Lucy*, Mac was "Ricky," and I was "Lucy," and that's how it remains to this day. We turned around and left. We ended up having done nothing in Manhattan except careen around the streets. We drove to the Short Hills mall in New Jersey, and that's the first time we "broke bread." He asked me if he should cut my food. "Is this my angel?" I thought. I had certainly experienced the devil in the very recent past.

Next thing I knew, no one could get in touch with me for two weeks. Everyone thought I was crying and pining for Nick Rick. Little did they know I was actually having a ball—with Mac!

On the third date, he told me that we were going to get married.

"That's stupid," is what came to my mind. But he was right because today, I'm Christine McCohnell.

The night before he left for Wyoming, he said, "I'm coming back to marry you."

"Okay."

He says he fell in love with me right then, and there I was thinking of Nick Rick, wondering if the nightmare would begin again. The day before Mac returned, Nick Rick showed up. What an asshole. I told him firmly that it was too late to rekindle our relationship.

On a different front, after the extremely hard work it took to defend my Disability Studies course at Ramapo (it was almost like a dissertation in a concise version), the proposal moved through three committees, and then I had to defend it to two other committees. Mike Fluhr was my number one supporter. Without his wisdom and helpful critique of my work, I would never have pulled this one off. It got approved the day after my thirtieth birthday. So this five-year mark turned out to be pretty good after all.

I vividly remember the day I found out that my course had been approved. I was sitting in Mac's kitchen, reading my email, and I screamed loudly, "Yay! It's been approved! It got approved!"

Mac's reaction? "What does that mean? Calm down."

Mac is a medical professional. He doesn't understand the academic field, and I don't understand the medical field. A perfect example of how our professional lives are so different: Mac would come home after a twelve-hour shift and I would greet him with, "How was work, honey?"

"Horrible. I had a cold." That's what I heard.

Being a sweet girlfriend, I made him chicken soup, and put some cold medicine on the table. He came back after taking a shower, and said, "What's this?"

"Well, honey, I thought you had a cold."

"No, I had a *code*." Meaning a patient of his died.

So you see how course approvals and codes can get mixed up and misunderstood at our house.

Mac and I had a courtship of three years. In May of 2004, we went to Chicago for five days, which was fantastic. We stayed at the Fairmont Hotel. I met his family, and I connected with them immediately. I met Mac's son (now my stepson), his wife, and their three-week-old baby, Mac's granddaughter. I held that darling baby and I started loving her right away.

Shortly after that trip, my mom, sister, and I took off for Italy for twelve unforgettable days. We went to exquisite Florence, but even before that, oh my God, the flight over there was a dream come true. I really don't know how my mother got my dad to fork over all that money for the three of us to fly to Italy first class. They even had an accessible restroom. I was in pure heaven. The seat turned into a big, comfy bed. We had outstandingly delicious gourmet food and fine Italian wine. We each had our own private movie screens with a zillion films to choose from. I brought some fun reading. I was literally in heaven.

When we got to Florence, it remained paradise. Not for the usual reasons, but because almost everything was accessible. Did you know that about Florence? Mom pushed me around everywhere, as I had not brought my scooter. Ah! Accessibility *and* no cars! It was so peaceful.

However, in the fine arts arena, my sister and I had completely different expectations. She wanted to see all the paintings, frescoes, and statuary of Florence, as most people do. Meanwhile, I said to myself, "These shitty pieces of work look exactly the same." Jesus and Mary were in almost every rendering. It was freakin' repetitive and I said so out loud, too. My sister was mortified. I'm sure most everyone else was mortified, too. I guess I had blasphemed.

I know that for most artists to make a living back then, they needed to be subsidized by a sponsor. That sponsor was often the Roman Catholic Church, and there were no competitors. Thus, the genius artists often rendered images of Catholic mythology. Yup, I said mythology. Almost all religions have their foundation built on mythology, whether it's Native Americans or any other indigenous tribe or the myth of Adam and Eve. Whew! I'm oh-so-politically incorrect here.

Don't get me wrong. Michelangelo's *David* and the masterful architecture of Firenze were amazing, but being so anti-Catholic, I really didn't enjoy seeing one ecclesiastic, Roman Catholic rendering after the other, after the other, after the other.

My idea of fun was watching the people outside the hotel. They were all so skinny, sauntering about. I also enjoyed talking to my mom about the meaning of life. Existential stuff outside religion, like "Who am I? Why am I? How do I belong?" We agreed on much more than I had thought we would.

After my trip to Florence, Mac introduced me, with great pride, to his brother and sister-in-law, Nicky and Brenda. They were so funny and nice. If Nicky likes you, he'll tease the hell out of you. By the end of the weekend we spent together, we acted just like brothers and sisters, and still do today. They know me so well that they even sense when I get mad at something without my saying anything about it. Everyone thought Mac and I made a great couple.

I wasn't totally crazy about Mac in the beginning, but in fairly short order, I knew I was gonna marry him and be in love with him for the rest of my life. My change of heart turned out to be only a few dates away.

As I approach our favorite Thai restaurant, I see his car. He wins again. Dammit.

Dating is not being married, right? I'm remembering our next date after the Manhattan adventure. We discussed our lives, like how we wanted to travel and see the world. We were both not in a hurry to get home that night. We strolled and relaxed in our new love. We held hands and didn't care about a thing in the world. The delicious conversation lasted for hours. When you're married, the conversation is so different. It's as different as night and day from puppy love talk. For example, as soon as I enter the restaurant this evening, it begins with the usual:

"Hello, Lucy. How was work, honey?"

"Shit. I was just thinking about the exams next week."

"Did you pay the bills today?"

"You know the carpet man is coming tomorrow to clean the house."

"I told you I had a doctor's appointment."

"Shit. I gotta get a gift for your Mom by tomorrow."

See how the conversation has shifted from sheer delight to dealing with everyday bullshit? I have to say, though, he always kisses me when we greet each other.

The staircase is absent from my mind. I have a career and a husband. My life is pretty calm, but you know me. Calm and I don't get along.

Up to 2003, nothing I had ever experienced in the dating arena resembled my courtship with Mac. Nothing even came close, including my addiction, Nick Rick. Mac was so calm. (I say that a lot, but it's true.) My parents said I had a glow on my face, and they were right. Still, with my track record, they were iffy about Mac. I'll never forget the first time my father met Mac. He told my dad that he was a vegetarian. In reply, my dad asked him if he was in a cult. I was mortified. It took several visits together before my parents grew to love Mac. And love him, they do.

When my uncle remarried, I attended the event with Mac. My aunts and uncles absolutely adored him. In fact, most people immediately adored him, but I hadn't. Now I do, yes, but I didn't at first. Why? I don't know, maybe because I had no reference point for a healthy relationship. I certainly love him with all my heart now. I'm married to him now, and I know his idiosyncrasies. Marriage is the hardest thing in the whole wide world, and when the marriage is good, it's all worth it.

Is it normal to question, "Did I marry the right man?" Then I look into his eyes and say, "Of course I did."

Is it normal to have a fight, and then three hours later, feel like shit because I love him so much?

I believe with all my heart that Mac loves me—because when I have a fight with him or throw a fit, all he does is play it off, then say *he's* sorry and make me laugh. But that pisses me off even more! I want to have a big argument, and he simply wants to keep me happy. His choice is always peace and tolerance. Live and let live. Lead by example.

I complained to my therapist about how, after my arguing with him, Mac turns around and makes me laugh. I can't believe how he does that! She replied, "The argument wasn't that bad because you forgot what you were arguing about. The problem you're experiencing is that your mom and dad did all their bitching behind closed doors. You always saw marriage as hunky dory. Sorry to say, kid, but it's not." I know better today what a healthy marriage is.

So, where was I before I started rambling on about an ideal marriage? Oh, yeah, I was telling you about our courtship.

During that time, Mac lived in Lebanon, Pennsylvania. The two-hour drive wasn't bad, but the people who lived there, I swear, were Jerry Springer-style guests. Not a lot of healthy lifestyles there.

You know how it is when you're dating--lovey-dovey. For example, Mac bought a beautiful backpack filled with wine and cheese. We had a fancy picnic, lounging on the grass next to each other. Now, after being married, we don't sit next to each other; instead, we sit across from each other so we can talk to each other better. Oh, and he almost never, ever even sips alcohol.

But back then in Lebanon, as he was whispering sweet nothings in my ear on our lovely picnic, I looked around the park and thought, "Can you believe this? The people here *really wallop* their kids!" I definitely felt like I was on the Jerry Springer Show.

After poor Mac realized that his sweet nothings couldn't compare with Jerry Springer, he gave up. He worked in a local hospital, so he was familiar with this atmosphere. I wasn't. You had wacky, unwashed people and crazy, local hillbilly people, all in one hospital!

I was falling in love for real this time. With Mac. It was so unlike any of the other men I was involved with. I'm probably confusing the hell out of you because I've had so many love interests entering and exiting my life. You may wonder, "Christine, how did you know that you were really in love this time?" Well, let me try to answer that. All the other men in my life wanted money—everyone except for Mac and my singing man (you remember Matt). Unlike the other men, Mac was health conscious and a teetotaler, and in due time, I was too. Well, almost.

I want to thank you for challenging me to probe life's questions and answers sincerely. In writing this memoir, I've realized that all the men in my life have been sexy, metaphorical answers to my emotional and physical needs, depending on where I was as I matured. Mac gives me security, peace, and stability. Nick Rick gave me an addiction. Fred gave me confidence, and I'm sure you remember what Ken gave me. All the other men were just occupying my time, even the one nerdy man in the bunch. (I'm laughing right now at my last statement.)

I love my husband, and he encourages me, even if it's against my will, to strive for the greater good, to attain difficult-to-achieve human and spiritual attributes (in other words, more Zen). Matt, for example, simply gave me pure love. More like a lazy river, and few goals for the future.

One week before my wedding, Matt came back to me via email, passionate as ever. He had no idea that my nuptials were right around the corner. Okay, Mac, please don't call the lawyer yet. The book's not over!

Back to Jerry Springerland in Pennsylvania. Rocky, Mac's brother, lives in Jerry Springerland Village. It puts me at ease to know that Mac has family just two hours away—even if it is in a wacky, hillbilly town. Rocky is a kind and gentle soul. My mother-in-law told me that when they were growing up, if you saw Mac, Rocky was two steps right behind him. We both love Rocky very, very much.

In November of 2003, Mac and I went to Orlando on a business trip for his company. We weren't engaged; we weren't married. Simultaneously, my parents had decided to visit Africa. Should I bother to tell my parents that I was in Florida? I was my own woman. I was successfully teaching First Year Seminar and my first Disability Studies class. One might ask, "Why should a professor be afraid of telling her parents?" I still thought of myself as their little girl--until June of 2006, when I got married. And believe it or not, I was actually too timid to tell them about my 2003 trip with Mac. I almost didn't recognize this timid version of me. I think all the Nick Rick shit had left me wary of telling anyone about my love life. This was understandable, considering all that had happened to me that year. Despite my furtiveness, my parents found out about the trip a month later when Mom saw a stunning, summery photo of Mac and me at Disney World. Oh well.

As the trips ended and we all returned to our respective residences, my sister was taking care of my grandmother because we all knew she wouldn't last very long. Kim had a lot of love for our grandmother, who lasted until my mom returned from Africa. My mom held my grandmother in her arms, in Grandma's own house, until she passed. Kim and I wrote the eulogy for the funeral. I still have it, because we never read it. Why not? Because my grandma always wanted everyone to be happy, and we were in tears. I'll tell you what though; my mom still carries that heartfelt eulogy in her wallet. And I honestly don't remember if most of the people were happy or not because it pains me to recollect the little I do. I'm weeping a bit right now

Isn't it funny how life plays out in the professional and personal arenas in our lives? Personally, I cried every day for a month about my grandmother. Professionally, my classes were the best ever. I had great kids. The first Disability Studies class was comprised of only seven of us. They all merited and received A's and one B+. I still remember their names and where they sat. Mike was right there in the class circle, too, arguing every point I was trying to make, just to piss me off! I don't know if he was doing this to make me know my academic material thoroughly, or if he was just doing it to add a little friendly confrontation. Either way, we entertained the students.

Christmas was hard for everyone, and I resented my father's mother, with whom I had little emotional contact, more than ever due to the fact that my "real" grandparents were dead.

That January of 2004, Mac moved from Jerry Springerland to Pottstown, PA. He hated it there. He had an eight-week assignment, and it was hell for him and me. The apartment that his agency gave him was small and in a dank basement. Pottstown was a poor, depressed town, and the apartment building's supervisor was straight from The Underworld. However, in the midst of all this, Valentine's Day was so special. We went to get massages, and then we dined at a great restaurant. It was the only good thing I remember about that time. Mac's company wanted to extend his time there, and he said, "Hell no."

During that same time period, we went back to Chicago to visit his family. It was delightful to see his son and granddaughter. The whole family was generous with us, and they sensed that something big was going on. Mac's next assignment was going to be more than four weeks in North Carolina, so they suspected that he'd propose to make sure all future "long term" separations would be lovingly bound by marriage.

I called my mom. "We're going to our favorite restaurant, and I think he's going to propose, and he better because I want a ring!" My mom had bought me a gorgeous jacket, which I was going to wear. She wished me good luck. Back at my future mother-in-law's house, people were whispering and chattering, taking pictures. I had the jacket on, too. No proposal.

"Okay, okay, maybe at the restaurant, and then we'll come back afterward. Okay, okay," I thought to myself.

The next thing I know, I'm in the airport, getting on a plane back to New Jersey! Shit, now what?

Later, my sister concluded, "The ring has to be somewhere in your house."

"Yes, I know! It's in the freakin' safe!"

"Well, can't we break into it?"

"No, Sherlock Holmes."

The night before he left for North Carolina, Mac and I were taking a nap together, and he announced, "Come on, let's go to dinner, so I can propose to you." How romantic is that? Plus, it was at a Thai restaurant--his favorite, not mine. Ugh. However, everyone at the restaurant knew he was going to propose. He got down on one knee and asked, "Will you be my soul mate for life?"

"Are you asking me to marry you?" I didn't know that's how Buddhists get engaged.

"Yes, Lucy, will you marry me?"

I cried and said, "Of course."

A big bouquet of flowers came out of nowhere. The whole restaurant knew, including the customers—everybody except me! Everyone smiled and applauded.

The next morning he left, and I felt as if he were going into the army. My parents were ecstatic. I didn't know this, but my mom had already been looking for places for our wedding for a month. How did she know? How did both my parents know? Intuition, I guess.

When Mac had initially brought up the subject of marriage, you wouldn't think that in this day and age, he'd have to ask my father for my hand in marriage. But that was the only way I'd have it. So that's exactly what Mac did. In my presence, he asked my parents for my hand in marriage. They said "yes," and of course, I said yes again.

Once upon a time, before I became engaged, my mom had said, "I don't know why people have engagement parties. That's so stupid." I wholeheartedly agreed, but when the subject of my own wedding came up, she changed her tune about engagement parties. Now she wanted one!

The day after Mac left, my sister took off from work and announced, "We gotta start looking for places for the wedding." My mom concurred, so we three went to several different places. One of them was horrendous; it smelled like mildew and we marched right out. We checked out the same place Charlie had had his reception. They had redone the whole place. It was beautiful, but to me it was way too fancy…it didn't feel like the right place. My mom wanted our wedding there so badly, but I said, "It's not homey. It's not for me." It was a typical high-class place.

The last place we looked at was the Summit Hotel. It was enchanting, simple, and my kinda homey. It had been a hotel since 1868. Horses and carriages had escorted patrons to the front door, and that lovely semicircle of an entrance still remained. In the twenty-first century, the historic atmosphere was beautifully in place, along with accessible, ADA accommodations. I knew, deep within my soul, that this was the perfect place. That night, we stayed in the Presidential Suite at the hotel. That sold *me*. Now I had to get the two important women in my life to agree or at least give their blessings.

Mom still wanted to have the reception at the "Swanky Suites" on a Saturday night—just like Charlie. I complained, "It's too much money, and, actually, it's pseudo-high class. It's tacky. Even if the Summit Hotel doesn't look like the typical wedding place, it's sweet and charming and perfect for the *relaxed* atmosphere *we* want." As you can see, I was not a typical bride-to-be. Actually, I was the complete opposite--I was super laid back. I also wanted it on a Sunday afternoon, so we wouldn't have to pay twice the price. Mom soon agreed with me.

Mom and I also differed on how many people were going to attend. Originally, my mom had wanted a wedding like my cousin's—fancy, black tie, Saturday night, with about three hundred people. I have to say, it was tempting to think of getting all that gift money, but, thankfully, we agreed on one hundred people, no black tie, and a Sunday afternoon.

Ever since I was a little girl, I had wanted to get married in my mom's back yard. I never understood why people spent so much money on one day. It's so much pressure. My mom declined, and we eventually compromised because my top choice had been to have the wedding at the house with only sixty people. We ended up with the reception *and* wedding at the Summit Hotel, which was truly lovely and unpretentious.

I will now entertain you with the components of planning our "simple" wedding.

First of all, it was a living nightmare. It wasn't about us; it was about everyone else. Still, my mom was the best wedding planner in the whole wide world. She shocked me when she told me we were having a big engagement party. When I reminded her of what she had said before, she retorted, "Well, I changed my mind."

Fortunately, the engagement party ended up being a big pool party. My dad made a speech, I made a speech, but Mac's speech was the best speech of them all.

I was told that before the engagement party you gotta have a date set for the wedding and know who's going to be in the bridal party. I didn't think that would be a big deal. Apparently, I was wrong.

Mac didn't care who was in the bridal party, so I sat down and really thought about it. If I were to ask one person, then I would have to ask another person. I ended up with ten bridesmaids and their escorts, plus a flower girl. That made twenty-one people, not counting bride, groom, and three of their parents. Holy shit. That would be more than one fourth of the wedding attendees. It was looking like a three-ring circus.

So I made a decision, and to this day I know it was the best solution. I had my sister as my maid of honor and my godchild as the flower girl. It was simple. Jamie, my godchild, always knew that when Aunt Christine got married, she would be in the wedding party. And it was obvious that Kim would be the maid of honor.

Simple, right? Hell no! Not in my family. I got hell from everyone. My cousin was so angry, and my friends felt hurt. My friend was hurt because I had been her maid of honor, and she wasn't going to be in the wedding party, at all. Denise was hurt, Trisha was hurt, every-freakin'-body was hurt. Even my sisters-in-law were hurt. There was only going to be a hundred people coming to this wedding anyway—so how many people could I put in the wedding party?! Ruthlessly, I stuck with my plan, and Mac stood by me. To make a long story short, my cousin and my aunt didn't even show up at the wedding because they were so angry.

My aunt had made the engagement period hell for me. As of Christmas of 2005, all ties were cut between my family and her family. I still feel guilty that my mom lost someone close over my wedding--my "simple" wedding. It remains one of my most painful memories. In a fury, she sent the invitation response back with a nasty letter. When I opened her card, as reminded of her mean words and actions all over again. I ripped up the check and dropped the gift off on her front porch before our honeymoon. It was horrible.

One of Mac's friends wanted to bring his kids. I said "No" because then everybody's kids would have to come! The friend said some unkind things to me, and I remember crying. Mac took the phone, and that ended *their* relationship.

Some invitees were not at all controversial, like the Stavitski's, their grown children, and my mom's friend from my preschool days, Lorraine, as well as her daughter, Tiffany. My pal Sandy from high school actually thanked me for not including her in the bridal party. So there!

The preparation for two souls uniting was not joyous at all, and this was supposed to be a happy occasion. Honestly, I just wanted to get the day over with and go on my damn honeymoon. I asked myself, "How can this be a joyous day with so much animosity surrounding a couple so much in love?"

Mac, as always, was calm and cool. True Zen surrounded by my family's tempest.

The seating arrangements were hell, also. The preparations continued to be a living nightmare. My friend Trisha had broken up with her boyfriend the week before. I was on the phone with her while she was crying and saying, "You should be happy. Your wedding day is tomorrow."

"Just another day."

But after all the traumas, my wedding day turned out to be perfect, absolutely perfect. I had no expectations, I didn't care, I thought it would be the day from hell. But it turned out be both spiritual and idyllic.

That morning when I woke up, something magical took over. I awakened in my old nursery. My mom came in with coffee and said, "Today's the day!"

I was surprised that my soul felt so good.

I was getting dressed when my dad came bounding up the stairs, calling out, "Teresa, you gotta see this." I shivered and thought that maybe my aunt had arrived. Instead, it turned out to be the largest, most colorful, magnificent butterfly we had ever seen. As Buddhists, Mac and I believe in reincarnation. (My conversion to Buddhism was born during my courtship with Mac. His Zen approach to everything always appealed to me, so I adopted Buddhism.) My maternal grandma had been so exquisitely beautiful on her own wedding day that I swear she was that very exquisite butterfly. She was there for me. She was awesome. The butterfly was there when I awoke and glided around the house until we got into the limo. It was she. I just know it. Everyone else may think I'm crazy, but let me believe what I want to believe on my wedding day.

Mom did my hair and my nails, and she had a woman come in to do my make-up. Kim and Jamie asked me, "How should we do our hair?"

"However you want, just like your pretty dresses you picked out."

Kim looked stunning, and little Jamie wanted two cute ponytails. I heard sly remarks about that later on. "How could Jamie just have two ponytails?"

I replied, "Because she wanted to."

On the ride to the hotel, I whispered in anguish, "When auntie shows up, what should we do?"

"Don't worry."

And I didn't. Thank God, she never showed up.

I remember sitting in the limo, watching people going into the hotel. Stevie came out and told me that Mac never showed up. Then he smiled.

"Don't mess with me. Is he here?"

"Yeah, I think so. Come on, let's go and get you married."

I looked at him and declared, "So he *is* here!"

Dad said, "Okay. Enough now." Just like old times.

My nieces and nephews handed out the programs I had designed.

We all lined up. My Nana and my mother-in-law walked in first. Then Mac's son (his best man) entered with Kim. Next, Jamie with her adorable ponytails was behind them. Then I walked in with my parents supporting me on either side. They kissed me and handed me over to Mac, my handsome groom.

As you can see, it was not your average church ceremony. Neither of us believed in church or synagogue or any kind of strict religious dogma. Clergy we contacted didn't want to take part in a nonreligious ceremony. One guy took a deposit, though, and scammed us. But the man who did marry us was the right one. He was a rabbi, and he married us in a large room at the hotel. He was the nicest man you'd ever want to meet. We met with him three times before the wedding. He didn't even want to take our money. His deep spirituality radiated.

We planned the ceremony the way we wanted it to be, from the very beginning to the very end. We even wrote our vows. Stevie and Nicky lighted the unity candles. Then my mentor, Mike Fluhr, read a poem. Mike had researched many poems in preparation, and the one he selected was, "Leap Before You Look." Several people later wanted to know what the hell that was. I knew, and Mac knew, and that's all that counted. Then, after "jumping the broom," we were officially wed.

Yes, I've mentioned that specific wedding/broom event before, but now I'll elaborate. I had asked my future mother-in-law what would she like to see on our wedding day. She jokingly said, "Jumping over the broom." We took it seriously, so each of us jumped over a broom. In slavery times in this country, when two slaves wanted to get married, they would jump over a broom to symbolize their marriage, because it was illegal for slaves to wed. Mac's last name, McCohnell, is associated with slavery because a family of slaves (Mac's ancestors) had taken on the Irish American name of their slave master. Mac's great-grandfather added the "h" and removed an "n" to identify more with families up north, where Mac's enslaved ancestors had fled via the Underground Railroad in the 1860s. There you have it: the real story to my new last name.

After the ceremony, we didn't have a receiving line because I thought it was stupid, and I didn't want to stand for that long. Jimmy, the maitre d' informed me that the bridal party would have a separate cocktail hour. For many weddings in New Jersey, this is traditional. He did not tell me that I would have the McDonald's version of the cocktail hour. We had shrimp, an antipasto platter, and pigs in a blanket. I discovered our guests enjoyed two rooms of sumptuous gourmet feasting!

We took pictures outside. It was a stunning day, one of the most perfect days of the year. They had me standing for over a half hour taking way too many pictures with family members and the bridal party. I needed a break, so I told the photographer, "I need to just sit down for five minutes, and then we can go on from there." That's when I noticed my guests walking around the hotel with huge shrimp, rack of lamb, and caviar, enjoying one of the finest five-star cocktail hours you'd ever want to have. My sweet mother-in-law tried to save a rack of lamb for me, and they told her she couldn't bring it into the banquet hall. But she said, "It's for the bride!" Well, till this very day, I never got my rack of lamb on my wedding day. I guess that's what I get for marrying a vegetarian.

After the photos, I was pooped, and the party hadn't even started.

I'm so glad that I had been strong-willed and had only my sister, my goddaughter, and my stepson in the bridal party. Their name announcements were mercifully brief. My mother-in-law did not want to walk in, so they just announced, "Julia McCohnell," and she smiled with big tears running down her face. Luckily, I didn't see that because I would have been crying hysterically. Next, my parents were announced, and of course Mom and Dad paraded in with pride and joy. Then everyone else stood, as Mac kept whispering to me, "Don't put your hand on your dress, you're going to get it dirty."

"Don't hold me that way. You know how to hold me." (Mac was holding me so that I could walk in without my walker.)

Jimmy smiled and said, "Welcome to married life."

We walked in as Mac was concentrating on keeping me upright, and I was waving and smiling to everyone. He kept saying, "Don't wave, you're gonna fall!" I didn't listen to him, and I didn't fall.

Our first dance was "The Love of My Life" by Brian McKnight. The song touched one of my friends, and she got it—no one else did. If you listen carefully to the lyrics, you'll probably have more insight than all the wild people at my wedding. Just listen to it, and do some emotional homework.

Next, my father and I danced to Rod Stewart's song, "Forever Young." That song held treasured memories for us. When I was little, my dad had an eight-track in the station wagon, and he used to croon Rod Stewart's songs to make me go to sleep. (Now how appropriate was that? Rod Stewart! Well, it always worked.)

Our terrific band consisted of twelve musicians, all African American. They were reputed to be the best band in New Jersey, and their silky name was Cashmere. The lead singer's voice was identical to Louis Armstrong, my mother-in-law's all-time favorite singer. She hadn't danced in thirty years, but she danced with Mac to their song, "How Wonderful You Are." It was amazing, purely amazing--a sincerely loving, spunky ninety-year-old woman dancing slowly with her beloved son. My stepson, the best man, was nervous and forgot to give a toast but still got up there and said, "I love my new Mom."

I said to Mac, "Oh my God! The toast—someone has to do the toast!" My oldest brother-in-law, who is never at a loss for words, gave a toast, and Mac's uncle's girlfriend said a prayer. Everything was great up till then. My father, in his former life, must have been a public speaker. His speech was fourteen minutes long! Fourteen! Have you ever heard of such oratory at a wedding? I wanted to throw a roll at him to shut him up. My aunt had a roll in her hand. I guess she was ready to fling it, too! He kept talking about his little daughter, but he rarely spoke about Mac. My aunt was about to get up and throw the damn roll, after all, but I think he saw her and finally ended the speech. Thank God for Aunt Gina. I was mortified and embarrassed, but everyone else, even

Mac, said it was the most beautiful, touching thing they had ever heard in their lives.

During his long speech, Dad claimed that I was the "Second Commander in Charge," and guess who was first? Take a wild guess! Mother Teresa! Even today, Dad still asks Mac, "How's the Second Commander doing?" Mac replies, "I bet just like the First Commander." Then they both laugh.

We had filet mignon and lobster tails. I told Jimmy I didn't like steak, and I wanted two lobster tails. Mac, who's a vegetarian, got eggplant Parmesan for his wedding. Jimmy bought out another two lobster tails for me. They were huge! My own Mother Teresa was cruising around, asking people, "You want another lobster tail?" She was doling them out. This was *not* a sophisticated wedding. Many happy guests devoured those leftover lobster tails.

The flowers were resplendent, everything was perfect, but true to form, I found it getting too stuffy. Then the band started up again, and they were not at all stuffy. Everyone was dancing, even my mother-in-law, who had vehemently declared that she'd never dance again after the slow dance with her son! Yessirree, she got up and boogied away. If I live to be ninety, I hope I have that much unbridled energy. What a treasure in our lives. In fact, for better or worse, both our families are treasures in our lives.

I was sipping my champagne out of a sterling silver straw because I can't drink without straws. I had forgotten about that essential detail, but my cousin soon reminded me during wedding preparations when she chimed in with, "You need a sterling silver straw at your wedding, you know." Slurping champagne through a straw made me a little tipsy, and Mac, the teetotaler, was tipsy, too.

After we had made the rounds of all the tables and thanked everyone, we put the envelopes with gifts in the specially designed festive birdcage. By then, with all these proprieties, it was too uptight for me. I challenged Mac, "I bet I can out dance you!"

"You know, this party is getting a little too formal. Let's have some fun."

I zoomed out on that dance floor with my husband, and we stayed there the whole night. Everyone was dancing with us. We even got the little kids up and danced with them. We drank wine on the dance floor, we made a big circle, and I made a big-ass mistake! Mac had to hold me up to dance, so during the ensuing dance competition between us, he cheated. When he got tired after a half hour of dancing with all the wedding guests surrounding us in a circle, I noticed his hand was letting go of mine. Looser and looser, and then I fell! Everyone at once said, "The wedding is complete because Christine fell!" Every wedding that I attend, I fall on the dance floor. It's a tradition, you know? When Christine falls, it's a sign that the bride and groom will have good luck.

But I vowed to make a swift comeback as an accomplished dancer. I promised to myself, "I'm not losing a competition to my husband!" When push came to shove, he beat me, because after another forty-five minutes of dance fever, his strong hands were barely holding onto mine, and down I went like a creampuff in my beautiful wedding dress. Cheater! Nonetheless, it was fun, fun, fun for me, the silly slipping bride, who also elected to not throw the bouquet or wear the garter. I didn't think that was necessary at our left-of-traditional wedding. We even cut the cake in privacy. Without a doubt, everything culminated in a great party where everyone had fun. Everybody celebrated the uniting of two souls, and that's what it's all about, anyway.

As the afternoon wore on, we boogied around and asked if people would dance with us some more, and if they wouldn't, I cracked a joke and twirled away. Trust me, a stuffy wedding becomes unstuffy once I get hold of it! My dress was falling down, my shoes were off, and I didn't care. I had my husband by my side. My walker was nowhere in sight the whole time because that day, we were one. Poor Mac. He was holding me up nonstop. In fact, almost everyone calls him, "Poor Mac," and it originated at our fun, festive wedding, heralded by extended families, best of friends, and co-workers. Mike Fluhr and other colleagues of mine were amazed that I could dance that well. My best friend's birthday was that same day, so we dedicated a song to her. Everyone joined in the good cheer, and just about everyone was getting tipsy. One of the best parts of the event was *after* the wedding when I heard all the stories about what had been going on. I could write a book on that!

I danced with him but once, and in times past, I usually danced with him all night long. Now he knows how I felt at his wedding. I would have preferred nondrunk.

At the end of the festivities, I was so tired. My sweet husband went upstairs to the suite and got the wheelchair because I couldn't walk anymore. No doubt about it, I had married the right man. Just as I was thinking to myself, "How the hell am I going to walk to my room?" out of nowhere the wheelchair appeared.

I'm always confused. You have this busy-ass day. You're so tired, you're so exhausted, and then you're supposed to do what you're supposed to do on your wedding night?! Sorry, Mom, we had already "done it" many a time; so it was not until the next night that we consummated our unity of souls. We later made up for it on our honeymoon, as well. Trust me on that one.

The next morning, I was still exhausted. Mac did the running around. He dropped off the wedding cake at my parents and did last minute things for the honeymoon, which weren't really necessary, but Mac had to expend some energy.

We honeymooned for two weeks in Barbados. Our island fairytale was not so different from the dream honeymoon I had wistfully yearned for as a little girl, when I had been captivated by the Bahamas. As it turned out, Barbados was wonderful. My parents' friends lived there for half the year and they were our unofficial travel agents, although we were not too interested in sightseeing, at first. They planned out the restaurants, the hotel, and the touristy stuff. For the first couple of days, we mostly did what honeymooners do, lots of passionate lovemaking. We hung out by the pool, ate breakfast on the patio, ate in the evenings at some really good restaurants, and later, took a tour around the island that consisted of very little to see. Aaaaaah. Relaxation . . . and being me, I got bored. It was a small hotel, so everybody knew us. The woman concierge asked on a daily basis, "How are the honeymooners, Mrs. McCohnell?"

I always gave her a great, big smile. But after a week I said, "I'm great, but I'm bored. Got any suggestions?"

Well, she did. She suggested that we go on a catamaran. We both agreed it was a fantastic idea. So, off we went onto the vessel. At the first stop, Mac and I agreed that he would check the water and see how safe it was to snorkel. Meantime, I would watch his wallet because there were about forty people on board with us. While he was snorkeling, the captain asked me if I wanted to go into the water. I said, "Sure."

Mac, who kept looking up at the boat, noticed what was transpiring and said to himself, "Isn't that nice, they're bringing Christine out to watch me snorkel."

The next time he looked up, Christine was in the water! He fumed to himself, "These guys probably make five dollars an hour, and my wife's life hangs in their hands. Come to think of it, that guy right there is feeling up my wife on my honeymoon!"

Mac is sometimes overprotective of me, but honestly, I didn't even think of it as a sexual thing I was just looking at a turtle, while the guys were "holding me up."

Mac swam over in a huff, and I chirped, "No, honey, you go snorkel. You go over there and have a good time. I'm having a good time right here. Plus, it's my turn to watch the wallet."

When we got back on the boat, Mac was quiet. He has never, ever yelled at me; when he gets mad, he just doesn't talk to me. Believe me, he didn't talk to me for the whole two hours back. But I knew I had messed up, and we made up.

A few days later, I got bored again. I suggested, "Let's go to a nightclub." But the nightclubs weren't air conditioned, and it was June in Barbados.

He bribed me: "I'll take you to the fanciest restaurant on the island. We don't have to go dancing in the hot weather."

Now do you see why he's called "Poor Mac"? He has to try to stay one step ahead of me. And I'm the one with CP!

So, I went with him to a fancy restaurant where all the celebrities had dined.

The next morning, I decided that I wanted to go jet skiing with my husband. He said, "I'm not going, but I'll pay the guy to take you." Mac finally realized what we had gotten ourselves into. He then declared that sort of thing would never happen again.

The rest of our honeymoon was spent relaxing with moments of his playing Ricky to my wacky Lucy.

Mac had orchestrated another romantic surprise for us on our honeymoon. He almost always thinks outside the box. He had asked the restaurant personnel if we could have dinner on the beach deck that evening. They replied, "No, Mr. McCohnell, we don't do that." But that very night there was a table set for two on the deck with a big bouquet and a jazz singer. Damn, I married the right man. I cried so hard they thought I was having a seizure. It was so beautiful walking up to the deck with the music and the ambience. At blissful times like that, I can almost forget the presence of the staircase of oppression in my life. Almost.

As we set out for home, we boarded the plane and the stewardess said, "You are in 1A and 1B." I looked up in surprise at Mac, and he said, "I love you, Mrs. McCohnell." We flew back first class, my favorite way to fly.

Our flight landed at 11:30 pm, so our friend Greg picked us up and brought us home. Mac wanted to carry me over the threshold. Instead, we decided to walk in the front door, holding hands as one.

I can't finish my Thai dinner. "I'm tired. I wanna go home, Mac. Let's not order dessert. I just wanna go to bed, I'm pooped."

"Okay, I'll get the check."

The romantic date from the past is almost absent from our minds. We are two loving and very exhausted people who want to hit the sack right now.

"Mac, could you turn off the lights?"

"Yes, Mrs. McCohnell."

And we kiss good night.

XXXXXXXXXXXXXXXXXXXXXX

The End and The Beginning

Epilogue

As I'm sitting here looking over the Disabled Parking Lot, I'm wondering, "Who is really disabled out there?" And then I think to myself, "Do I have the authority to judge anyone?"

Oh, I forgot to tell you it's been three years since our honeymoon. Quite a bit has happened during those three years. As I said, I'm sitting in my office, writing to you once again, for closure for you and for me.

Mac and I are still at Zen Farms with the greenery that we cherish every day. Mac is now working at an institute for people who have CP. I am still at Ramapo College, teaching Disability Studies and overseeing the development of a new Disability Studies minor at the college—it will be the only one in the state.

I'm also on the board of the Society of Disability Studies, and the chair of the annual SDS conference. So on a professional note, we are a busy couple dedicated to our careers.

As for the families, those branches on the tree that never go away, they're still there: Mom and Dad are traveling the world, Stevie is free of cancer and now recovering from a hip replacement, Charlie is still Charlie, but I love him and he knows that, Kim is special to my heart. Can you believe that Kelsi going to college in two years? My godchild,

Jamie, with the big brown eyes, has her own cell phone—God, kids are lucky today!

CJ is the cutest thing I've ever seen. If I don't see him for a month, he says "I miss you, Aunt Christine" and he sits on my lap. Mind you, he's 10 years old! How sweet is that…and I hope he sits on my lap when he's 16 and his girlfriend is right next to me!

Nina is full of questions and wonders why Uncle Mac and I are different; she wants to help us. She's a very sweet and gentle soul, but she'll beat anyone at T-ball. My Stevie had to tell her, "Now don't beat up those boys!" "Okay, Daddy. Maybe just one?"

Jason and Nevaeh still play a big part in our lives because they are our immediate family even though they live in Chicago. My mother-in-law is still funny and as lively as ever—still telling her jokes. The other day she told Mac, "I'm falling off the bed!" I said, "Mom, we can't have that!" She replied, "I better whisper when I joke!" You gotta love my mother-in-law, and I do love her so much. Come to think about it, she substitutes for my beloved Grandma and I am grateful.

I often wonder about the pile of leaves. Some leaves are still on the branch and it's not for me to say who they are. But the one thing I have to say, the pile gets bigger and bigger. The leaves are blossoming more than ever in our life now. I truly hope I brought a little wisdom to your soul.

This epilogue is dedicated to Mike Fluhr. Thanks, Mike, for everything. I wouldn't be writing this epilogue in my own office without you.

I think that's it…until next time…be good, or at least try, anyway!

www.ingramcontent.com/pod-product-compliance
Lightning Source LLC
Chambersburg PA
CBHW061302280526
45784CB00002B/859